FITNESS *for* WOMEN OVER 60

The information contained in this book is not intended and should not in any way replace the direct relationship doctor-patient or specialist examination.
It is recommended to always seek the advice of your doctor and/or specialists regarding any indication reported.
The publisher and the author do not guarantee nor assume responsibility for the information in any form.

Author: Liam King

Art director: Thomas Baglioni

Graphic design: Lisa Albizzati
www.lisaalbizzati.com

Independently published

First edition, october 2021

ISBN: 9798757149868

FITNESS *for* WOMEN OVER 60

Reverse The Aging Process With Simple Exercises to do at Home or Outdoors, Regain the Strength, Endurance, And Energy You Had 10 Years Ago in 4 Weeks

Elizabeth Foster

Table of content

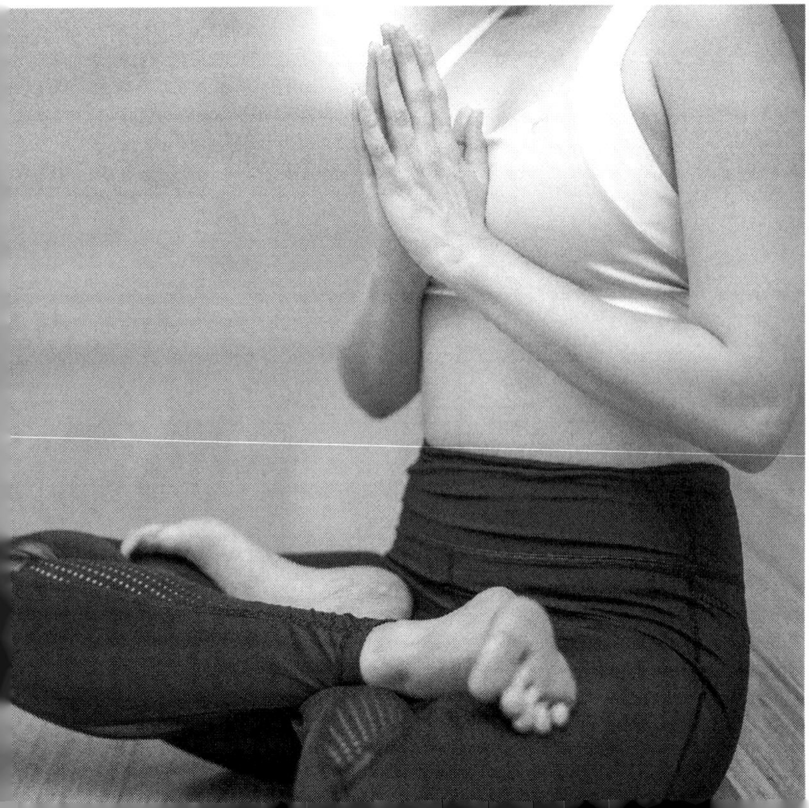

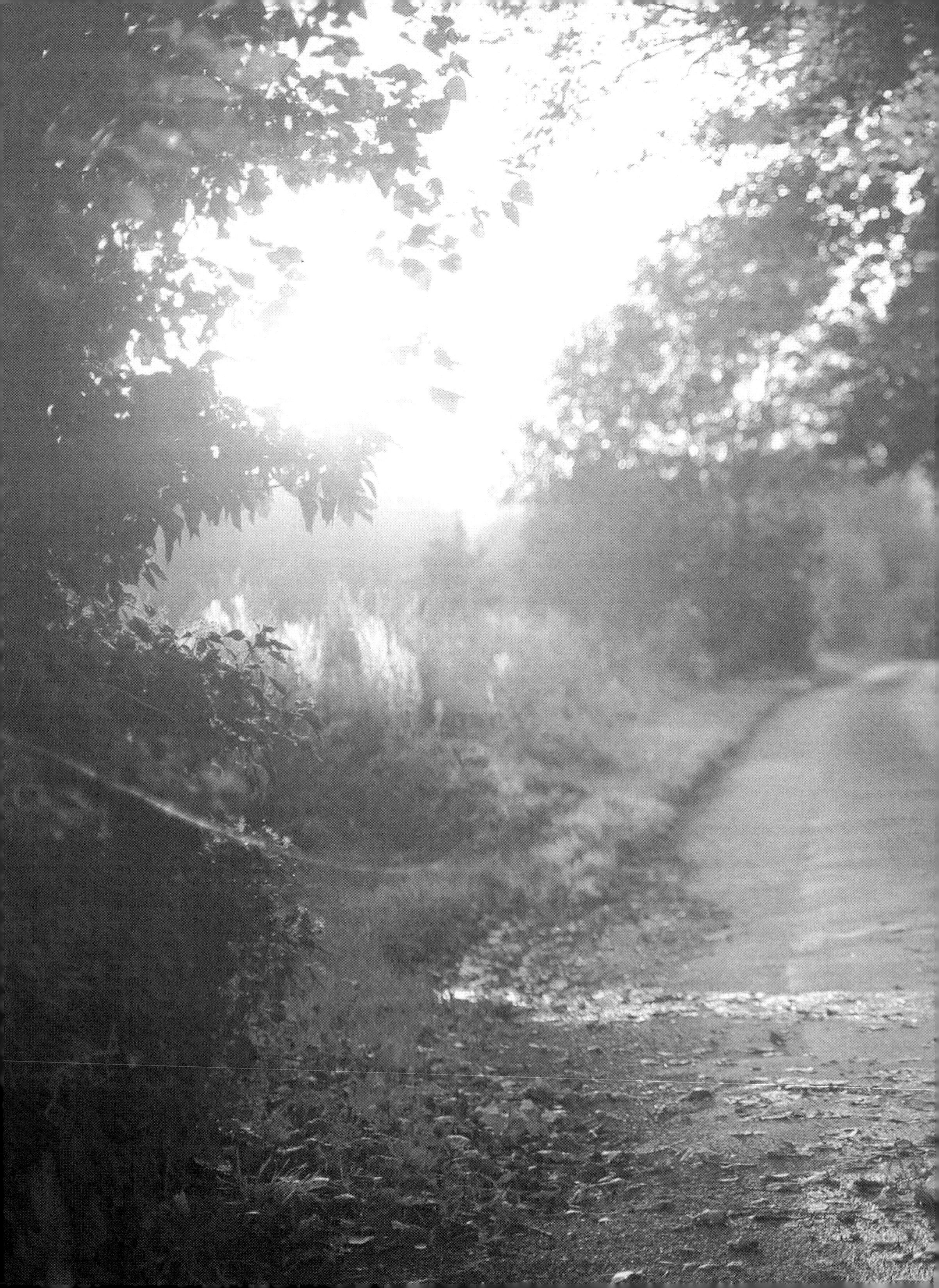

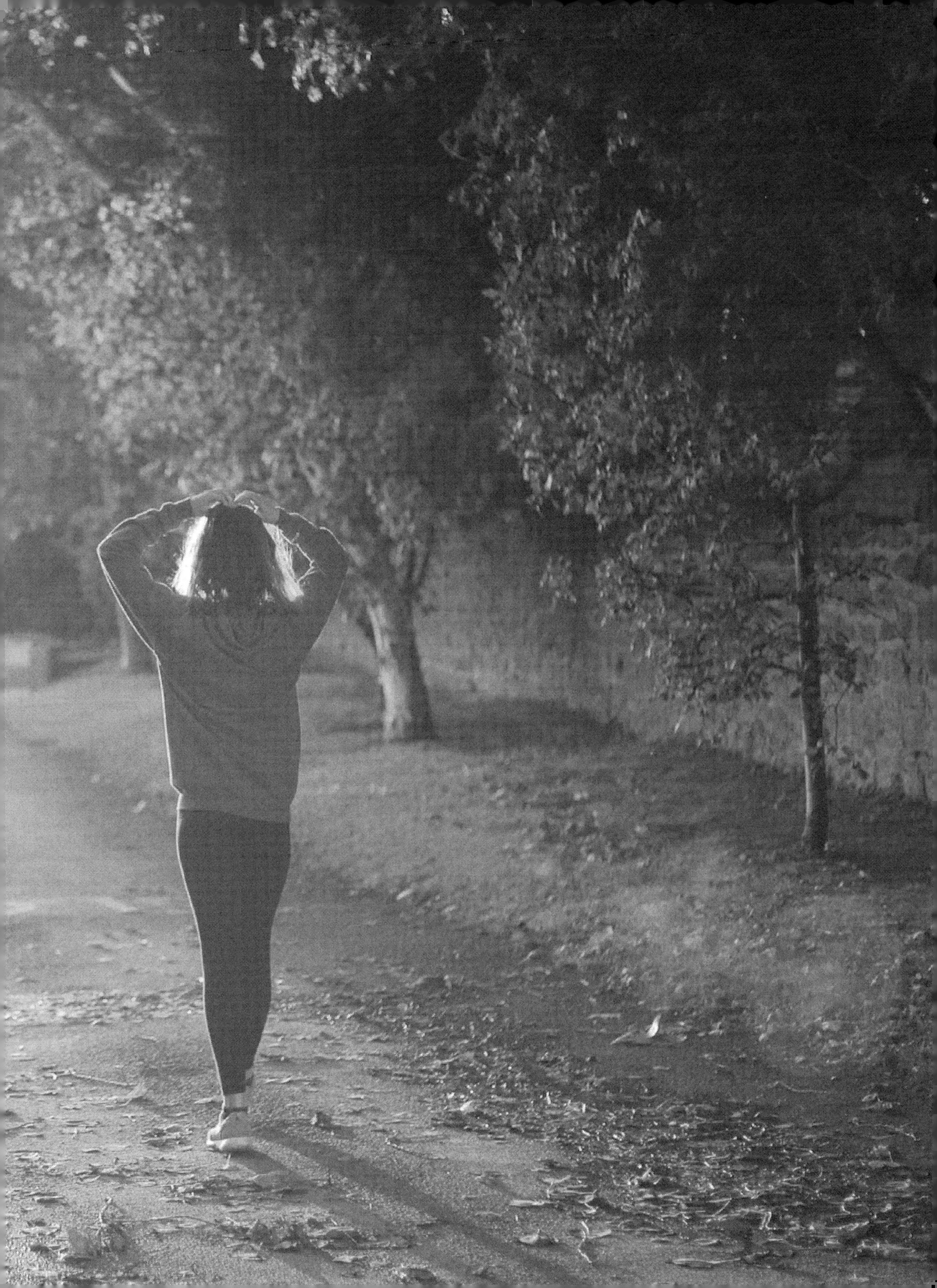

Introduction

Once you are over the age of 40, the aging process is inevitable.
With it comes a set of changes in your body, your mind, and your lifestyle. That means it's time to take action if you want to stay healthy and vital.

Although there is no denying that it's easier for an 18-year-old woman to maintain her strength and muscle tone than it is for a 70-year-old, strength and muscle can be maintained and even improved throughout life.
That's the good news. The bad news is that your body changes as you age.

The post-menopausal years are particularly challenging because hormone levels change significantly during this time of life. Many of these changes are beneficial, including slower metabolism, less muscle mass, less body fat, and fewer injuries due to decreased flexibility resulting from the loss of connective tissue.

According to the statistics, over 60% of elderly women do not engage in regular physical activity. In addition, many of these women remain sedentary both during leisure time and at work.
However, because this age group has been at a relatively high risk for cardiovascular issues and other health-related problems due to low levels of physi cal activity, it is important for them to engage in some form of exercise or strength training regularly.

In order to ensure your well-being as you grow older, be sure that you include a minimum balance of moderate aerobic exercise and strength training in your regimen each week. Just make sure you incorporate these types of moves into your daily workouts—which will provide the added benefits mentioned above.

When you are physically active, you'll improve your overall health tremendously. Not only that, but it will also help you feel more energized throughout the day. Look into the following benefits of regular physical activity to keep in mind as you target healthy aging.

Regular aerobic exercise is good for your mental health and lowers stress levels, which will allow you to enjoy your life more. This is especially important as you age so that you can combat feelings of loneliness and isolation.

Heart health is another benefit of regular physical activity—especially strength training exercises if they are done correctly. Strength training exercises engage your heart, arms, and legs while simultaneously working out several muscle groups at once. This results in faster rates of oxygen uptake to the muscles, which improves cardiovascular health.

Strength training will also help tone the abdominal muscles and other muscle groups. This will decrease your risk of falls and give you more flexibility with your joints. The more muscle you have, the more calories you burn during your workouts. This will also help reduce your body fat percentage at the same time. Not only does physical activity result in weight loss, but it can also improve bone health and overall health. Regular strength training exercises work on raising calcium levels in the bones so that they are not as susceptible to osteoporosis later on.

Physical activity can help you prevent cognitive diseases that affect the brain, such as Alzheimer's and dementia, in older adults. Regular physical activity helps improve your mood and combat feelings of anxiety and depression in older adults.

There are also benefits of physical activity that are directly related to your mental health, including being able to handle stress better later in life.

Physical activity is an important part of slowing down the aging process due to the amount of improvement it provides. However, even though it can improve your well-being and overall health, not everyone should start strength training exercises at this age.

Cardiovascular health is very important for older adults as it can be vital in preventing strokes—one of the leading causes of death for senior citizens. Physical activity and strength training exercises help improve cardiovascular function and reduce the risk of heart disease and high blood pressure, which can be very common issues. Most importantly, regular physical activity will help your heart work more efficiently, resulting in a longer lifespan.

This book will focus on the benefits of strength training exercises for older adults, as well as how to incorporate them into your weekly workout routine without sacrificing your health.

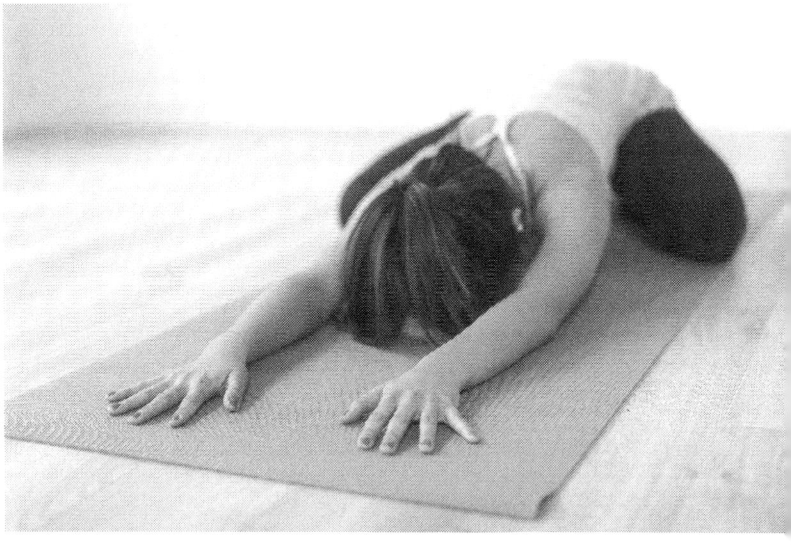

Exercises to Increase Strength

Doctors recommend having at least 150 minutes of physical activity a week. Spread out over the week. That's 30 minutes of activity for five days. Workouts are great, but you'll have to give your body time to adjust and recover. Two days of rest and recovery can be inserted midweek or during weekends. From 150 minutes, you'll build up to 225 minutes, and eventually 300 or more minutes a week. These routines aren't set in stone. As you progress and learn and get used to the exertion, you'll have the confidence and the personal knowledge to mix and match exercise moves you feel would best suit your body's strength and endurance levels.

Beginner Fitness Level

Here's a sample stretching, strengthening, and cardio routine.

3 minutes of warm-up stretches.

- Perform 2 times, Upper Back Stretch
- Perform 2 times, Chest Stretch
- Perform once on either side of the neck, Neck Stretch
- Perform 2 times, Sit and Reach Stretch
- Perform once for each leg, Inner Thigh Stretch
- Do 1 set of 16 reps, Shoulder Circles
- Do 1 set of Hand Stretches

8 minutes of muscle-strengthening and balance exercise.

DAY 1

- 2 sets of 16 reps, Seated Shin Strengtheners
- 2 sets of 8 reps, Pliés
- 2 sets of 10 to 15 reps, Front Arm Raise
- 2 sets of 5 reps for each side, Side Bends
- 2 sets of 8 reps, Tummy Twists
- 2 sets of 10 repetitions for each hand, Wrist Curls
- 4 sets of 15–20 steps, Toe the Line
- 2 sets of 10-second Flamingo Stands for each leg
- Perform 3 Clock Reaches for each side

DAY 2

- 2 sets of 10-second Flamingo Stands for each leg
- 2 sets of 10 repetitions, Side Leg Raise
- 2 sets of 10 to 15 reps, Front Arm Raises
- 2 sets of 5 reps for each side, Side Bends
- 2 sets of 8 reps, Tummy Twists
- 2 sets of 10 repetitions for each hand, Wrist Curls
- 2 sets of 10 to 12 reps, Bicep Curls
- 2 sets of 16 reps, Seated Shin Strengtheners
- 2 sets of 8 reps, Pliés
- 2 sets of 10 to 15 reps, Wall Push-Ups

DAY 3

- 2 sets of 5 reps for each leg, Leg Lifts
- 2 sets of 15 reps, Seated Knee Lifts
- 2 sets of 10 repetitions, Knee Extensions
- 2 sets of 10 to 15 reps, Front Arm Raises
- 2 sets of 10 repetitions for each hand, Wrist Curls

- 2 sets of 10 to 12 reps, Bicep Curls
- 2 sets of 16-second Single Limb Stance with Arm for each leg
- Perform 3 Clock Reaches for each side
- 2 sets of 8 to 10 reps, Modified Burpees
- 2 sets of 5 reps for each side, Side Bends
- 2 sets of 15 reps, Seated Twists

DAY 4

- 2 sets of 5 reps for each leg, Leg Lifts
- Perform Bicycles for 30 seconds, rest, then go another 30 seconds
- 4 sets of 15–20 steps, Toe the Line
- Do 2 turns on the Speed and Agility Drill ladder
- 2 sets of 10 repetitions for each hand, Wrist Curls
- 1 set of 10 reps, Dumbbell Upright Row
- 2 sets of 10 to 15 reps, Wall Push-Ups
- Perform 3 Clock Reaches for each side
- 2 sets of 8 to 10 reps, Modified Burpees
- 2 sets of 8 reps, Pliés
- 2 sets of 16 reps, Seated Shin Strengtheners

DAY 5

- 2 sets of 10-second Flamingo Stands for each leg
- 2 sets of 16-second for each leg, Single Limb Stance with Arm
- 2 sets of 16 reps, Seated Shin Strengtheners
- 2 sets of 8 reps, Pliés
- 2 sets of 5 reps for each side, Side Bends
- 2 sets of 8 reps, Tummy Twists
- 2 sets of 15 reps, Seated Twists
- 1 set of 10 reps, Dumbbell Upright Row

- 2 sets of 10 to 15 reps, Wall Push-Ups
- 2 sets of 8 to 10 reps, Modified Burpees

15 minutes of cardio exercises.

5 minutes marching in place.

10 minutes of brisk walking.

ALTERNATE CARDIO A

- A 15-minute bike ride or

ALTERNATE CARDIO B

- 5 minutes of easy resistance on a stationary or elliptical bike
- 10 minutes of medium resistance on a stationary or elliptical bike
- 2 minutes of cooldown stretches
- Perform 2 times, Upper Back Stretch
- Perform 2 times, Chest Stretch

Perform the cooldown routine below:

March in place for 30 seconds.

You should feel a bit of a stretch on your left calf. Hold the position for 16 counts. Switch positions and repeat step number 2 with your left leg.

Step your right foot behind and rest your hands on your right knee. Slowly bend from the waist, pushing your buttocks backward and up.

You should feel a bit of a stretch on the back of your left thigh muscles. Hold the position for 16 counts. Switch positions and repeat step number 4 with your left leg.

March in place for 60 seconds. Stand with a wide stance and spread your arms upwards to stretch. Sweep your arms down to the side and raise them up again. Repeat this move for 8 counts.

The routine above is a sample for those with beginner-level fitness who scored below average fitness test results. This routine should be done for two weeks to get the body and muscles limber before attempting the fitness test again. Always remember to do warm-up exercises before doing more strenuous movements. Cooldowns are also important to help your body recover from the exertion of the physical activity it just experienced. Always have water on hand when exercising. Keep hydrated throughout by drinking before you start and especially after you're done with your routine.

Remember to pace yourself before progressing to the next fitness level. You're competing with anybody but yourself. The goal is to achieve your desired fitness goal, and this is a marathon, not a race. People respond differently to exercise. Your results are uniquely yours. Don't compare your pace and progress with that of others. People's bodies respond differently based on current health conditions and prior exercise experience. The important thing is to keep going.

Vary the routines using any combination of moves that you'd like to do. Remember the proportion of cardio to strength training exercises: 70% and 30% for beginner level, 60% and 40% for intermediate level, and 50% and 50% for expert level. Start with 2 sets and increase the number of sets and repetitions when you've gained strength and confidence in executing the moves. Warm-up and cooldown routines don't have to be changed. Its purpose is to loosen and relax muscles to avoid strain. Never skip out on doing warm-ups and cooldowns.

You noticed in the routines set above. The changes are in the cardio and strength exercises. If the movements are too many to follow or keep track of, you can focus on three or four that you can repeat and cycle through for the duration of the strength training routine. Remember to keep proper form. Don't rush through your routine. It's a surefire way to get injured and hurt yourself. Pace yourself and rest for 15 seconds before making the next move.

Intermediate Fitness Level

The next set of routines are for someone with an intermediate fitness level. You're doing great! Four weeks in, and you're making great strides with your health, and your physical strength is showing improvement. Each routine is 45 minutes long and has more lifting involved and varied cardio exercises. The equipment you'll be using for these exercises would be easily adaptable and substituted with common household items. Weights don't necessarily mean more dumbbells or barbells. Instead, you'll use your body weight. A note about adjusting the number of reps and sets: if you can go longer without fatiguing your muscles, you need to add more weights to build strength and mass. Fatigue should be a good kind of sore. Stop what you're doing if you feel any pain or discomfort.

The routine and exercises set out here are alternated—more exercises and longer reps on some days and three or four moves repeated in decrements of 50, 30, and 20 seconds on other days. Always remember to take 15-second rests before transitioning to the next move or set.

3 minutes of warm-up stretches.

- Perform 2 times, Upper Back Stretch
- Perform 2 times, Chest Stretch
- Perform once on either side of the neck, Neck Stretch
- Perform 2 times, Sit and Reach Stretch
- Perform once for each leg, Inner Thigh Stretch
- Do 1 set of 16 reps, Shoulder Circles
- Do 1 set Hand Stretches

15 minutes of muscle-strengthening and balance exercise.

DAY 1

- 2 sets of 20-second Flamingo Stand for each leg
- 6 sets of 20 steps, Toe the Line
- 3 sets of 15 reps, Front Arm Raises
- 3 sets of 16 reps, Seated Shin Strengtheners
- 2 sets of 8 reps, Pliés
- 1 set of 10 reps, Partial Squats
- 1 30-second Modified Plank with a box or a chair
- 3 sets of 12 reps, Bicep Curls
- 2 sets of 10 repetitions, Dumbbell Upright Row
- 2 sets of 10 repetitions, Knee Extensions with resistance bands
- 3 sets of 8 reps, Tummy Twists
- 3 sets of 10 repetitions, Modified Burpees
- 1 20-second Wall Sit
- Perform 4 Clock Reaches for each side

DAY 2

This exercise routine has fewer moves, but longer reps and more sets and will be repeated 3 times. Make the moves with as many reps as you can, or hold the position for as long as you can for 50 seconds for each move or exercise on the first round.

- Do a Flamingo Stand for each leg
- Pliés
- Partial Squats
- Modified Plank with a box or a chair
- Wrist Curls
- Dumbbell Upright Row
- Front Arm Raises
- Modified Plank with a box or a chair

Repeat and cycle through the moves a second time for 30 seconds for each move and 20 seconds for the third round.

DAY 3

- 2 sets of 20-second Single Limb Stands for each leg
- Perform Bicycles for 30 seconds, rest, then go another 30 seconds
- 3 sets of 12 reps, Bicep Curls
- 2 sets of 10 repetitions, Dumbbell Upright Row
- 1 20-second Wall Sit
- 1 30-second Incline Push-Ups with a box or a chair
- 3 sets of 12 reps, Forward Step-Ups
- 2 sets of 10 repetitions, Side Bends
- 2 sets of 10 repetitions, Seated Twists
- 3 sets of 8 reps, Knee Extensions with resistance bands
- 3 sets of 10 repetitions, Modified Burpees
- 1 20-second Wall Sit
- 1 set of 10 reps, Partial Squats

DAY 4

This exercise routine has fewer moves, but longer reps and more sets and will be repeated 3 times. Make the moves with as many reps as you can, or hold the position for as long as you can for 50 seconds for each move or exercise on the first round.

- Do Clock Reaches for each hand and side
- Tummy Twists
- Side Bends
- Dumbbell Upright Row
- Seated Knee Lifts
- Modified Burpees

- Wall Sit
- Modified Plank with a box or a chair

Repeat and cycle through the moves a second time for 30 seconds for each move and 20 seconds for the third round.

DAY 5

- 3 sets of 16 reps, Seated Shin Strengtheners
- Perform Bicycles for 30 seconds, rest, then go another 30 seconds
- 3 sets of 10 repetitions, Modified Burpees
- 1 30-second Modified Plank with a box or a chair
- 3 sets of 12 reps, Bicep Curls
- 2 sets of 10 repetitions for each hand, Wrist Curls
- 2 sets of 10 repetitions, Dumbbell Upright Row
- 1 20-second Wall Sit
- 1 30-second Incline Push-Ups with a box or a chair
- 6 sets of 20 steps, Toe the Line
- Do 2 turns on the Speed and Agility Drill ladder
- 3 sets of 15 reps, Front Arm Raises
- 1 set of 10 reps, Partial Squats
- 25 minutes of cardio exercises.

ALTERNATIVE CARDIO A - Walking and Stair-Climbing

- 5 minutes of marching in place
- 5 minutes of Forward Step-Ups
- 5 minutes of kick-backs, sidesteps, and front kicks
- 5 minutes of marching in place
- 5 minutes of Lateral Step-Ups

ALTERNATIVE CARDIO B - Speed Drills and Stair-Climbing

- 5 minutes of marching in place
- 5 minutes of Speed and Agility Drills
- 5 minutes of kick-backs, sidesteps, and front kicks
- 5 minutes of marching in place
- 5 minutes of Step and Stand Speed Drill

ALTERNATE CARDIO C - Bike or Cycling

- 5 minutes of easy resistance on a stationary or elliptical bike
- 10 minutes of medium resistance on a stationary or elliptical bike
- 5 minutes of high resistance on a stationary or elliptical bike
- 5 minutes of easy resistance on a stationary or elliptical bike
- 5 minutes of cooldown stretches
- Perform 2 times, Upper Back Stretch
- Perform 2 times, Chest Stretch

Perform the cooldown routine below:

March in place for 30 seconds.

Lunge forward, taking care not to let your knee go over your toes.

You should feel a bit of a stretch on your left calf. Hold the position for 16 counts. Switch positions and repeat step number 2 with your left leg.

Step your right foot behind and rest your hands on your right knee. Slowly bend from the waist, pushing your buttocks backward and up.

You should feel a bit of a stretch on the back of your left thigh muscles. Hold the position for 16 counts. Switch positions and repeat step number 4 with your left leg.

Stand and hold on to a wall for support. Keep your standing leg slightly bent to avoid strain. Hold the position for 16 counts.

You'll feel a bit of a stretch on the front of your thighs. Alternate with the other leg and perform the stretch 2 times for each thigh.

March in place for 60 seconds. Stand with a wide stance and spread your arms upwards to stretch. Sweep your arms down to the side and raise them up again. Repeat this move for 8 counts.

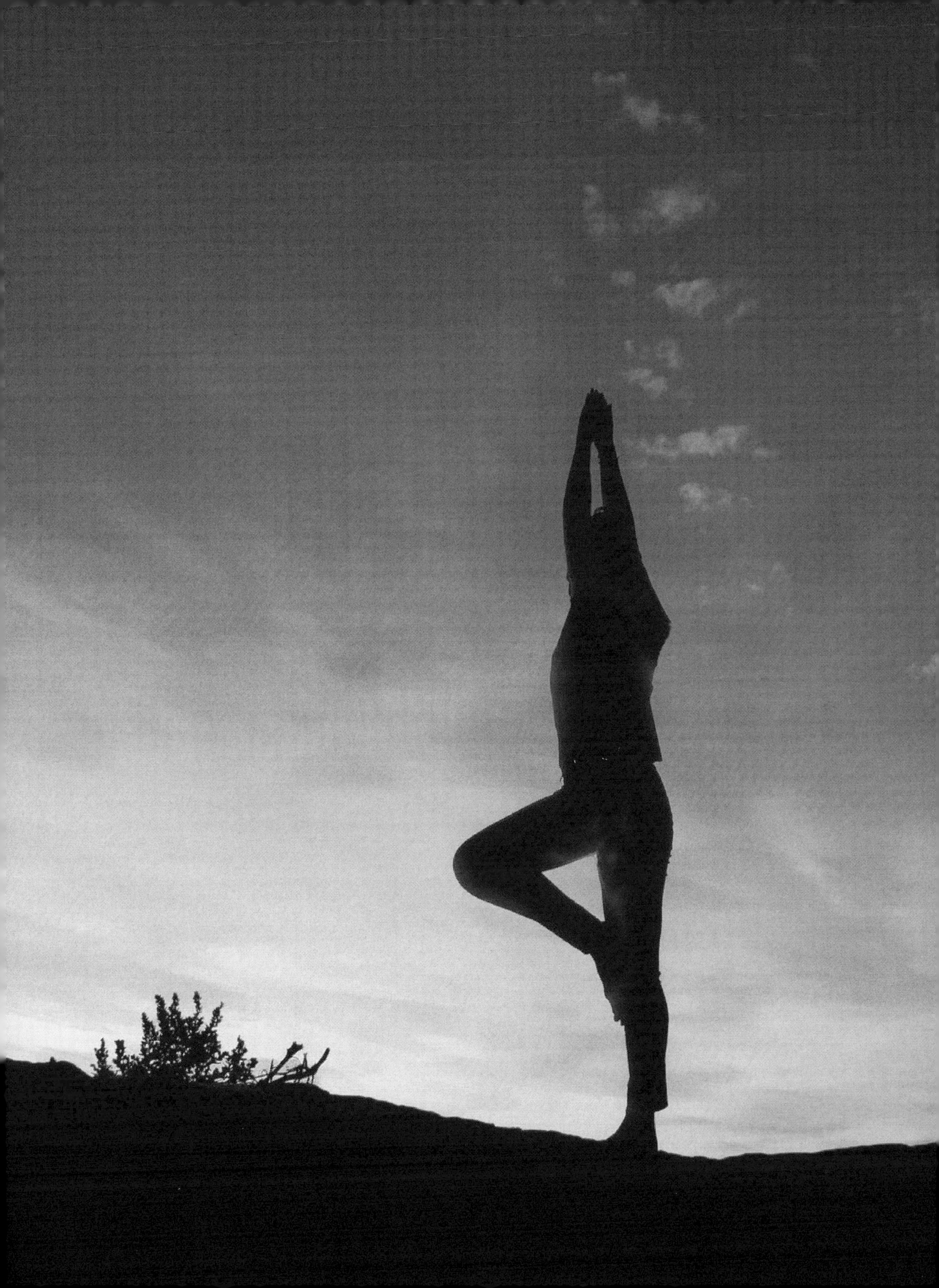

Chapter 1: **Exercises to Increase Endurance**

Week 1

Day 1

Total Workout Time: 30 Minutes

Exercise	Reps	Sets	Rest
Air Squats	10–15	2	90 Seconds
Triceps Dips	10–15	2	90 Seconds
Swimmers	10–15	2	90 Seconds
Glute Bridge	10–15	2	90 Seconds
Press Ups	10–15	2	90 Seconds
Dead Bug	10–15	2	90 Seconds
Standing Toe Touches	10–15	2	90 Seconds
Cow	30 seconds	2	90 Seconds

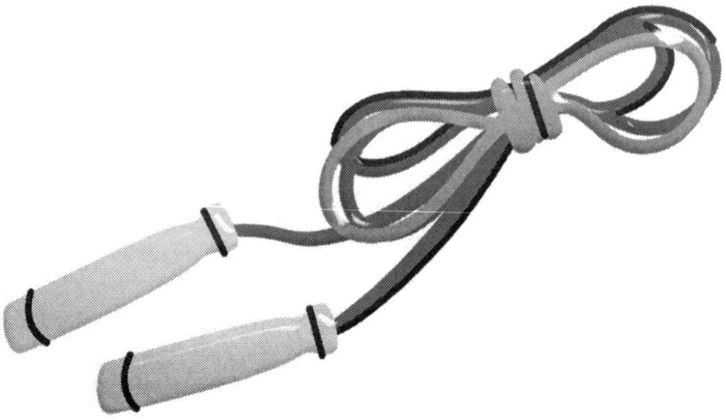

Day 2

Total Workout Time: 30 Minutes

Exercise	Reps	Sets	Rest
Deadlift	10–15	2	90 Seconds
Bird Dog Plank	10–15	2	90 Seconds
Clams	10–15	2	90 Seconds
Hollow Archs	10–15	2	90 Seconds
Long Lunge	10–15	2	90 Seconds
Hammer Curl	10–15	2	90 Seconds
Boat	10–15	2	90 Seconds

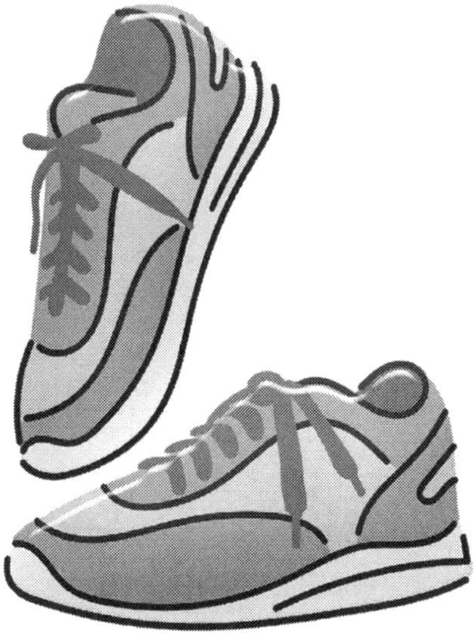

Week 2

Day 1

Total Workout Time: 30 Minutes

Exercise	Reps	Sets	Rest
Plié Squat	10–15	2	90 Seconds
Split Stance Row	10–15	2	90 Seconds
Donkey Kicks	10–15	2	90 Seconds
Leg Raises	10–15	2	90 Seconds
Single Leg Box Squa	10–15	2	90 Seconds
Shoulder Press	10–15	2	90 Seconds
Reverse Lunges	10–15	2	90 Seconds
Sphinx	30 seconds	2	90 Seconds

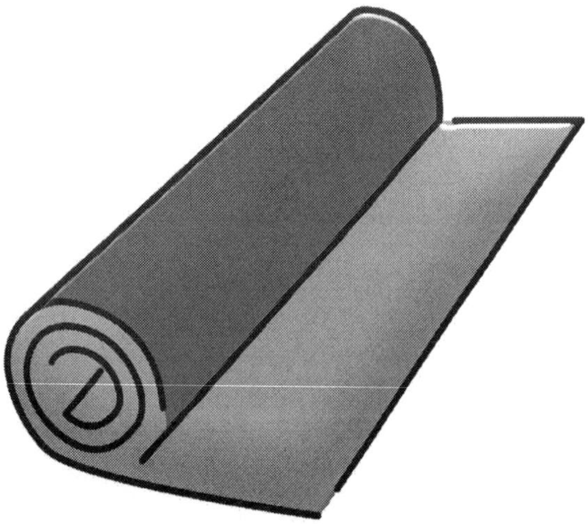

Day 2

Total Workout Time: 30 Minutes

Exercise	Reps	Sets	Rest
Single Leg Raise	10–15	2	90 Seconds
Lateral Raises	10–15	2	90 Seconds
Side Lunges	10–15	2	90 Seconds
Cat Cow	10–15	2	90 Seconds
Knee to Elbow Extension	10–15	2	90 Seconds
Shrugs	10–15	2	90 Seconds
Wide Squa	10–15	2	90 Seconds
Cobra	30 seconds	2	90 Seconds

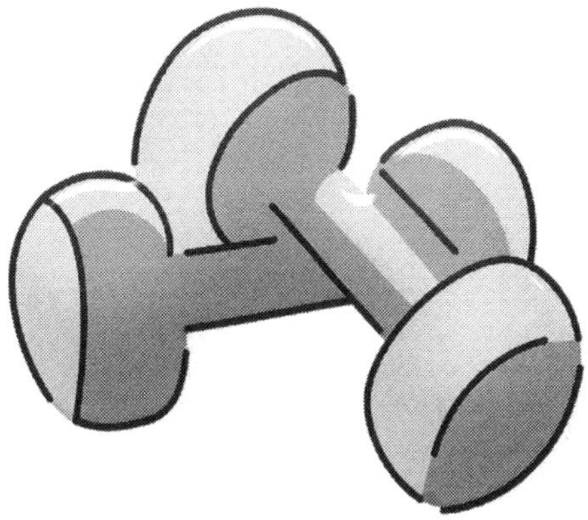

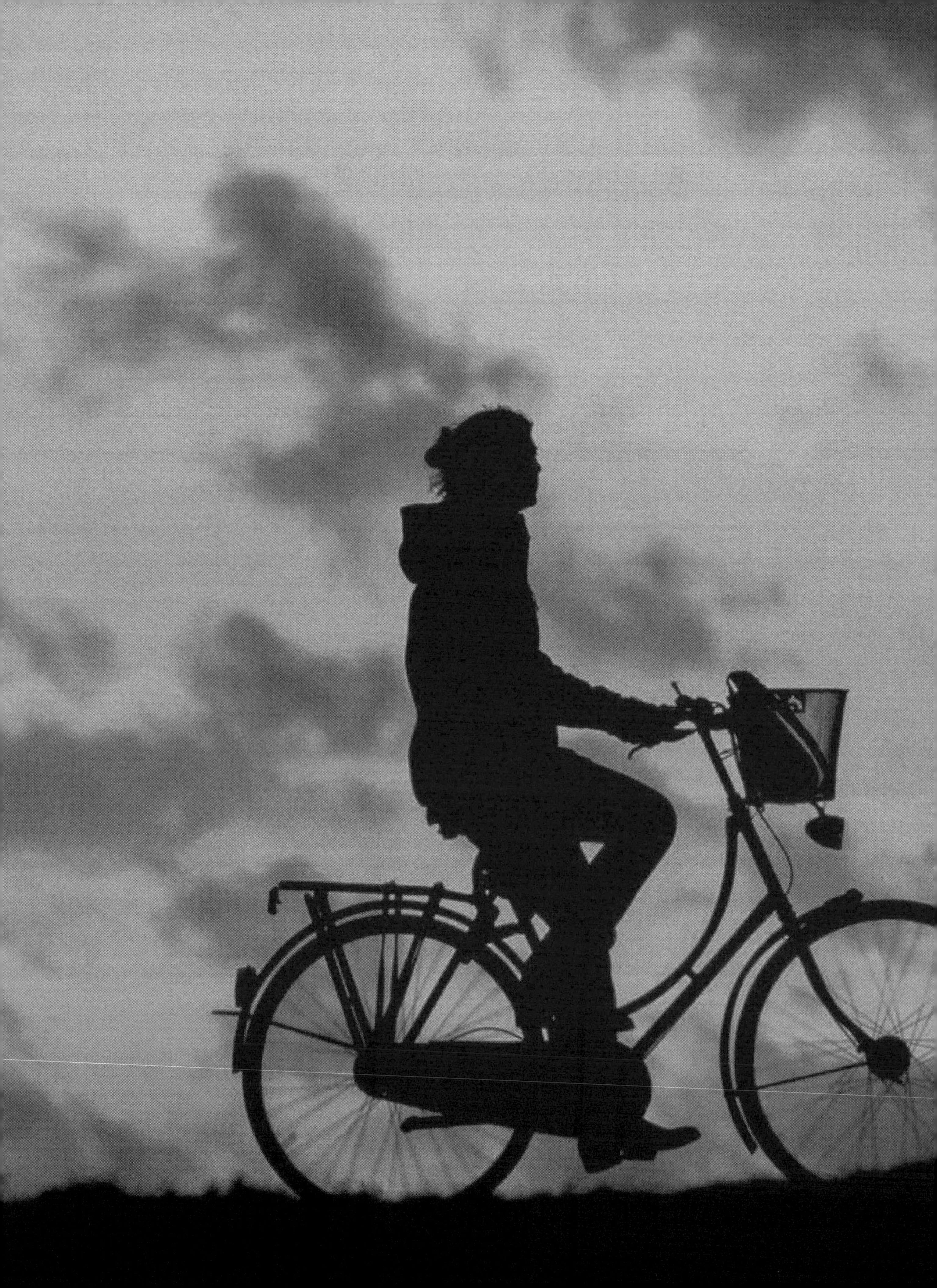

Air Squats

Air squats are a multi-joint exercise working your leg muscles, including the glutes, quads, hamstrings, calves, and core. Squatting is needed for a range of everyday tasks, from standing up from your chair to picking something up off the floor.

Instructions:

1. To perform the air squat, stand with your feet shoulder-width apart.
2. Keep your back straight and core engaged throughout the exercise.
3. Drive through your mid-foot to return to standing.
4. During extension, push your knees out.

Tip: When setting up for the air squat, "screw" your feet into the floor.

Easier Option: Lower your buttock ¼ of the way down, rather than below your hips.

Harder Option: Add weight or add a jump during extension.

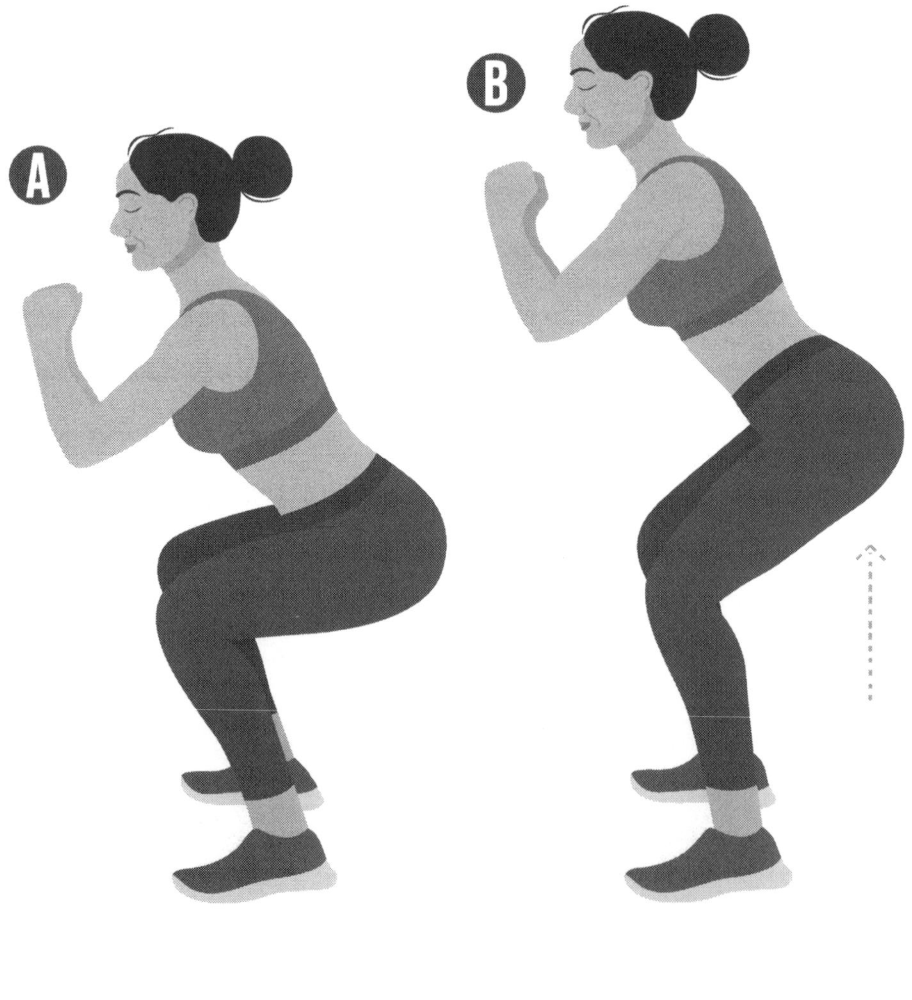

Triceps Dips

Triceps dips are an upper body exercise focusing on the backs of your arms. Our triceps help us extend our arms.

Instructions:

1. To perform a triceps dip, you'll need a raised surface such as a chair or a bench.
2. Bend your elbows until they form a 90-degree angle, then push through your palm to return to extension.

Tip: Look forward rather than down at your feet to keep your neck in a neutral position.

Easier Option: Bring your feet closer to the elevated surface.

Harder Option: Move your feet further from the elevated surface.

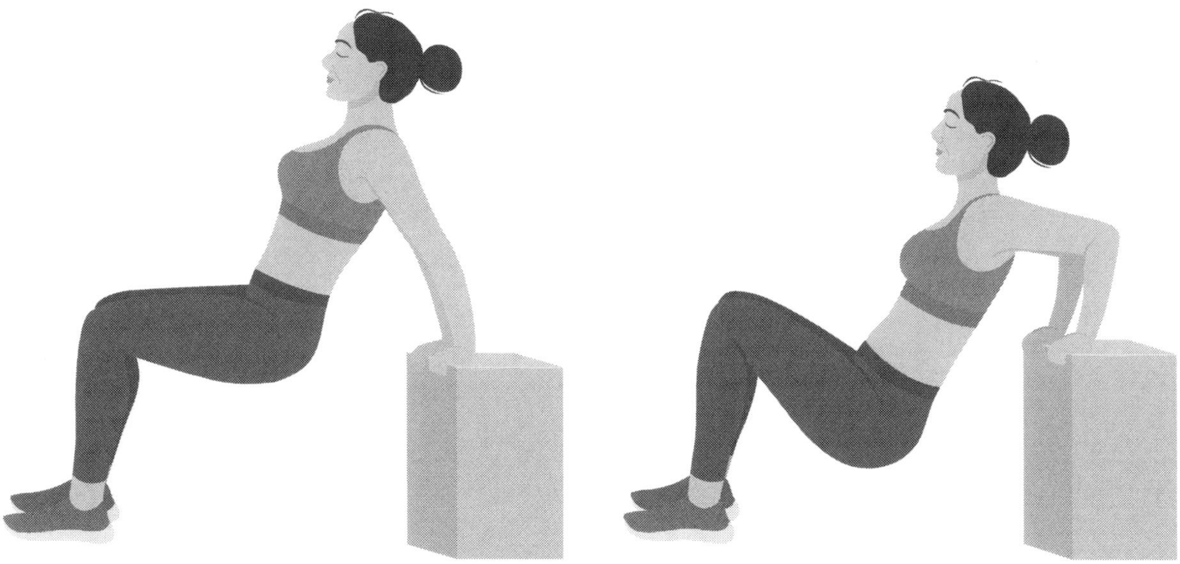

Swimmers

Swimmers are an advanced version of alternating superman; they work single limb strength and stability in your upper back, lower back, glutes, hamstrings, and core.

It's a great exercise for improving posture and alleviating back pain.

Instructions:

1. Begin lying face down with your legs extended and arms above your head.
2. Push your hips into the floor while squeezing your core and buttocks.
3. Lift your arms and feet off the floor slightly—this is your starting position.
4. Lift your right arm and left foot as far as you comfortably can.
5. Lower to the starting position while simultaneously lifting your left arm and right foot.

Tip: Think of the action like a front crawl.

Easier Option: Perform alternating superman.

Harder Option: Hold a weight in each hand.

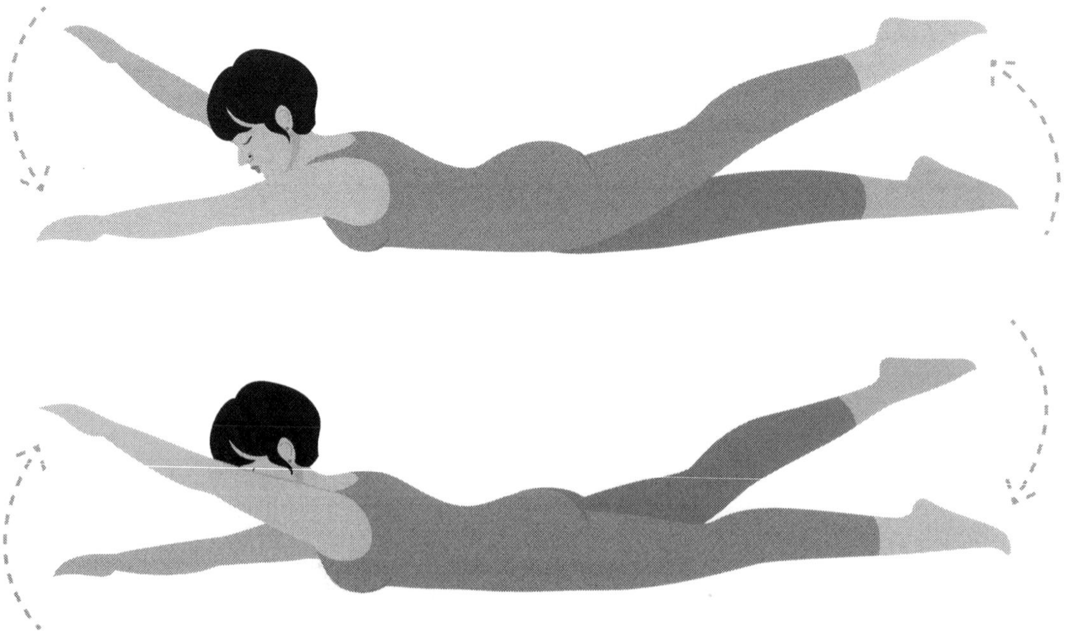

Glute Bridge

The glute bridge works the glutes, core, lower back, hamstrings, and hips. The glute bridge can also be used to alleviate knee and lower back pain

Instructions:

1. Pull your feet to your buttock until they are flat on the floor.
2. Push your shoulders, upper back, and lower back into the floor while squeezing your core.
3. Engage your glutes, then push your hips towards the sky.
4. Pause at the top for two seconds before slowly lowering.

Tip: Push your knees out during extension.

Easier Option: Place your feet further from your core.

Harder Option: Place a weight on your groin area.

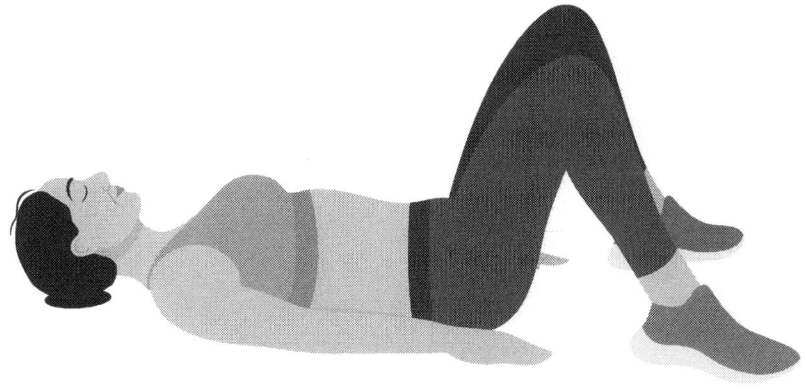

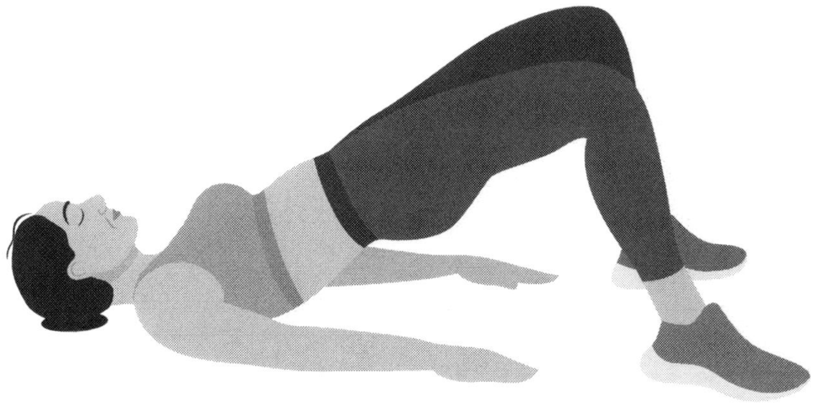

Press-Up

The press-up is one of the best bodyweight exercises for building upper body pushing strength. It helps build strength in the chest, shoulders, triceps, biceps, and back. It also helps strengthen the shoulder joint.

Instructions:

1. Start in the plank position.
2. Place your hands under your shoulders and toes on the floor.
3. Your shoulders, buttock, and ankles should all be aligned.
4. Squeeze your core and buttock.
5. Bend the elbows to lower your chest to the floor.
6. Pause for one second before pushing through the palms to return to the starting position.

Tip: Your hips and shoulders should move together. Don't bend your back to make the movement easier.

Easier Option: Perform the press-ups on your knees.

Harder Option: Pause for four seconds at the bottom of the push-up.

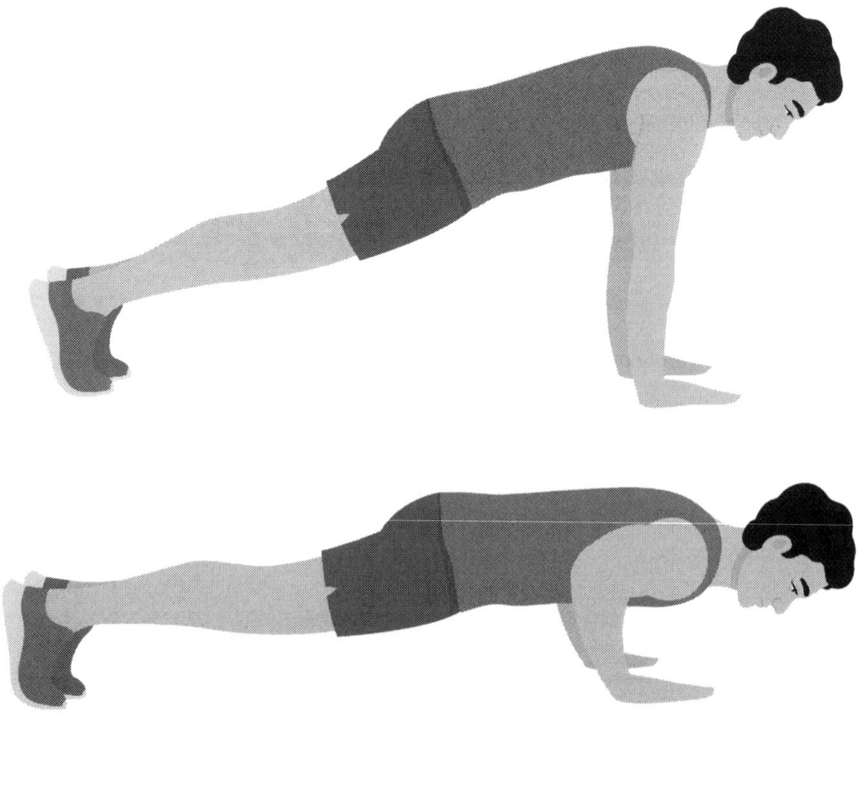

Dead Bug

Dead bugs are a core exercise to help develop your core strength, coordination, and balance. They're great for strengthening the smaller muscles in your shoulders and hips too.

Instructions:

1. To perform the dead bug, begin by lying face-up on a mat.
2. Bring your knees towards your chest at a 90-degree angle and extend your arms towards the ceiling.
3. Slowly lower your right arm and left leg towards the floor.
4. Stop about 1-inch above the floor, pause for a second, then return to the cen ter before repeating on the other side.

Tip: Press your lower back into the floor to engage your core.

Easier Option: Only move your leg or arm, not both.

Harder Option: Hold a weight in your hands.

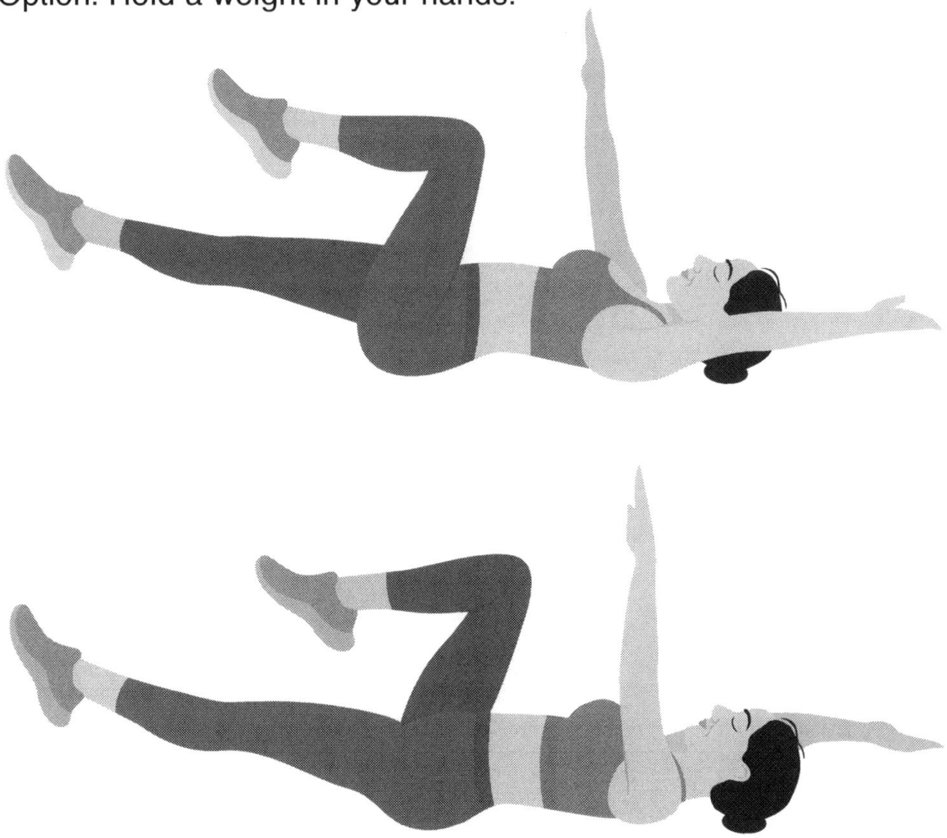

Standing Toe Touches

Standing toe touches are a great exercise to improve your mobility, core, and leg strength. It predominantly works your obliques and hamstrings.

Instructions:

1. Stand tall with your feet shoulder-width apart.
2. Keeping your legs straight, raise your right leg in front of you as far as you comfortably can.
3. Meanwhile, raise your left arm to meet the toe.
4. Slowly lower and repeat on your opposite side.

Tip: Keep your core and glutes tight.

Easier Option: Bend your knees slightly.

Harder Option: Hold a weight in each hand.

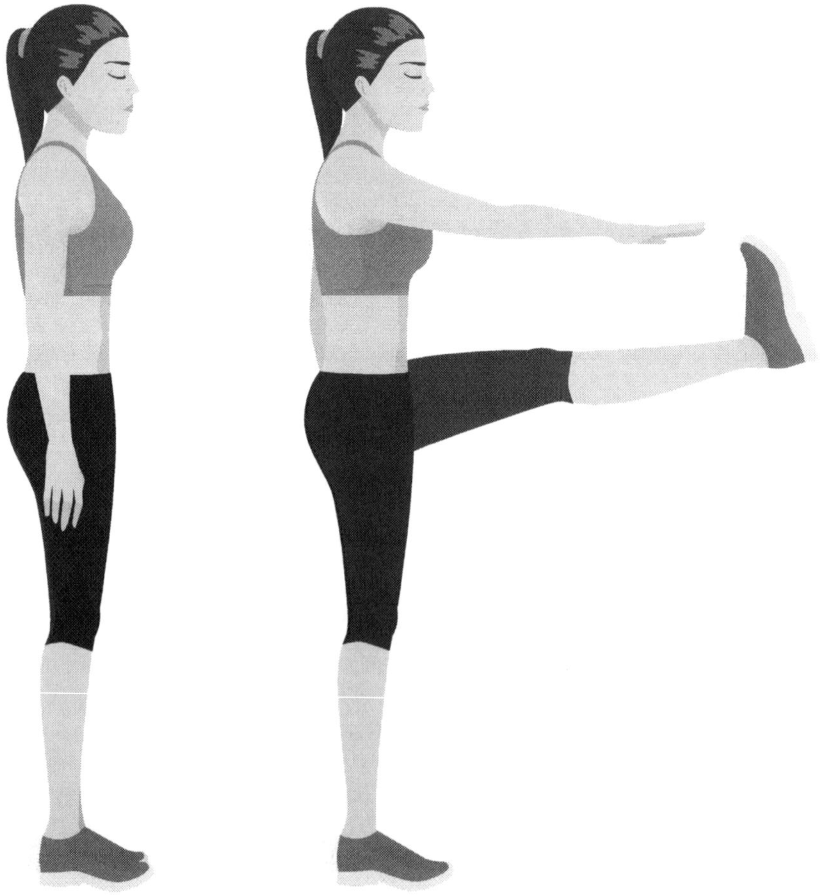

Cow

The cow is a yoga pose that stretches your torso and neck. It's a great way to improve your posture and spine health.

Instructions:

1. Begin on your hands and knees.
2. Ensure your hands are directly under your shoulders and knees under your hips.
3. Keep your head in a neutral position and squeeze your core.
4. Lift your chest while drawing the belly button down.
5. Hold this position.

Tip: Pull your shoulder blades apart and down.

Easier Option: Release the position every 10 seconds.

Harder Option: Perform the cat-cow exercise.

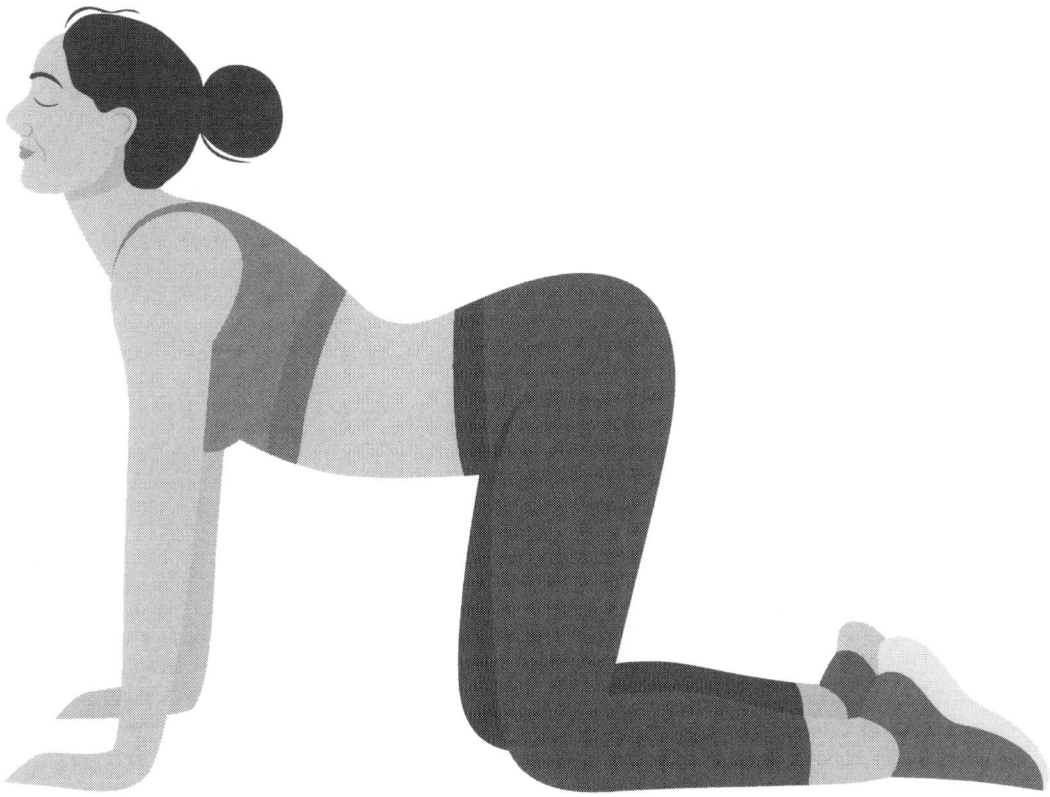

Deadlift

Instructions:

1. Begin standing tall with your feet hip-width apart.
2. Hold a weight in each hand at your sides.
3. Pull your shoulder blades together and engage your core.
4. Send your hips back, then bend at the knees.
5. Lower the weight as far as you can without rounding your back.
6. When you've reached maximal depth, push the hips forward to return to standing.

Tip: Keep your neck in a neutral position by looking at a spot on the floor in front of you.

Easier Option: Perform the exercise without weights.

Harder Option: Perform the deadlift with a barbell to reach greater depth.

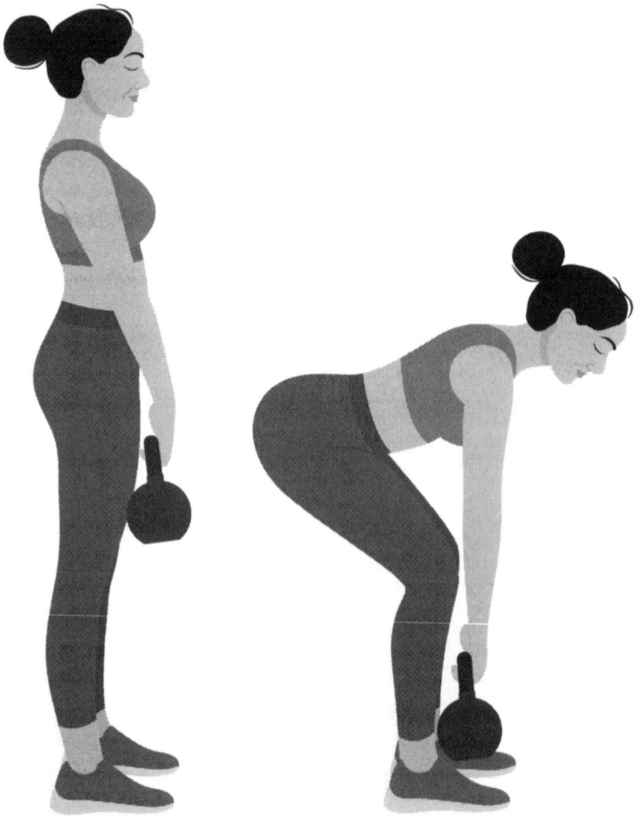

Bird Dog Plank

The bird dog plank improves full-body stability and strengthens your spine, back, core, glutes, hamstrings, shoulders, and triceps. Transferring your weight onto single limbs is a great way to build joint strength and control.

Instructions:

1. Start in the plank position.
2. Place your hands under your shoulders and toes on the floor.
3. Your shoulders, buttock, and ankles should all be aligned.
4. Squeeze your core and buttock.
5. Extend your right leg and left arm until they are parallel to the floor.
6. Hold for two seconds before returning to the starting position.
7. Repeat on the opposite side.

Tip: Practice shifting your weight onto your arms before getting your legs involved.

Easier Option: Raise your legs only.

Harder Option: Hold for five seconds at the top of the movement.

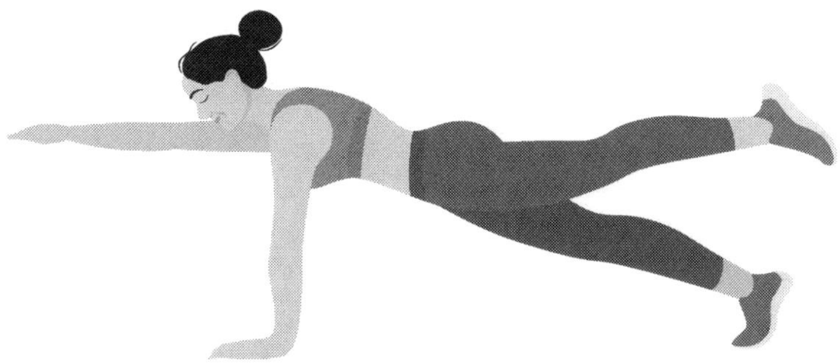

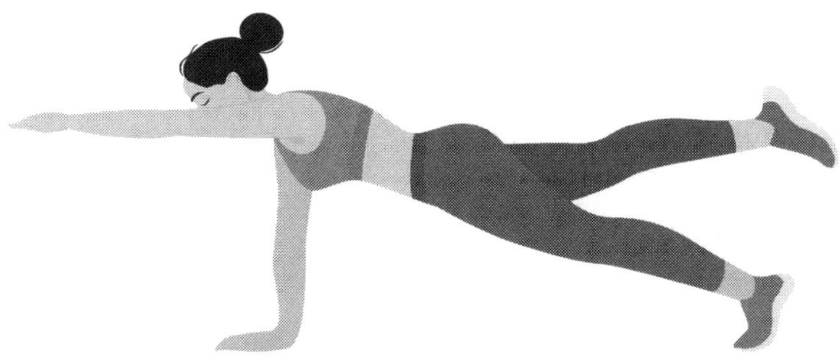

Clams

Clams build strength in the glutes, inner and outer thighs. Your glutes play a significant role in stabilizing your pelvis. Therefore, it's important we keep it strong.

Instructions:

1. Begin lying on your left side with your hips and shoulders aligned.
2. Bend your knees slightly and prop your head up with your hand.
3. Brace your core and tuck your belly button in.
4. Keeping your toes together, rotate your right knee as far as you can without breaking hip alignment.
5. Pause for two seconds before returning to the starting position.

Tip: Keep your neck still.

Easier Option: Reduce the range of motion.

Harder Option: Wrap a resistance band just above your knees.

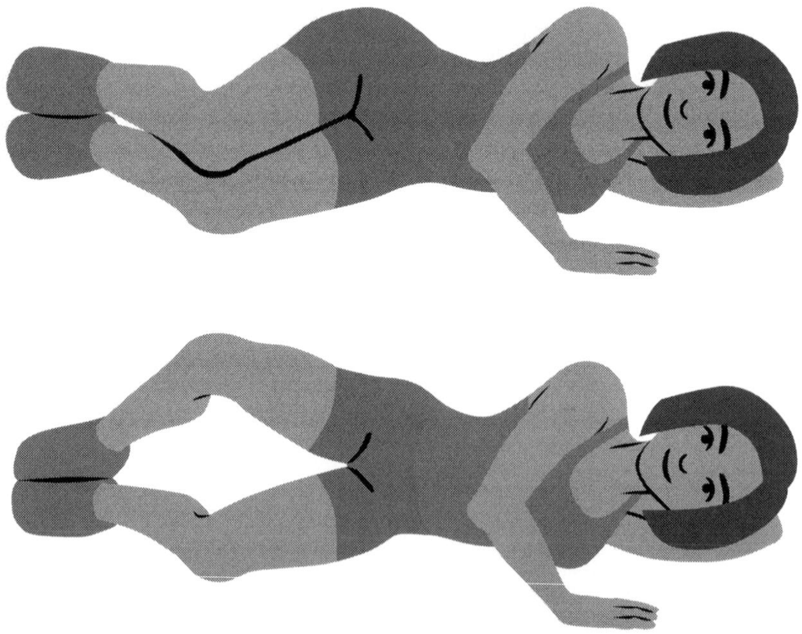

Hollow Arch

Hollow arch helps build a strong and stable core. They target the abdominals, diaphragm, hip flexors, and core. They are also beneficial for improving your posture.

Instructions:

1. Begin lying on the floor with your legs extended and your arms above your head.
2. Push your shoulders, upper back, and lower back into the floor while squeezing your core.
3. Squeeze your ankles together and arms to your ears.
4. Lift your upper back and feet off the floor until you feel your abs tense.
5. Hold for a second before slowly lowering.

Tip: Keep your lower back pressed into the floor through the exercise.

Easier Option: Only raise your feet, not your upper back.

Harder Option: Hold a weight in each hand.

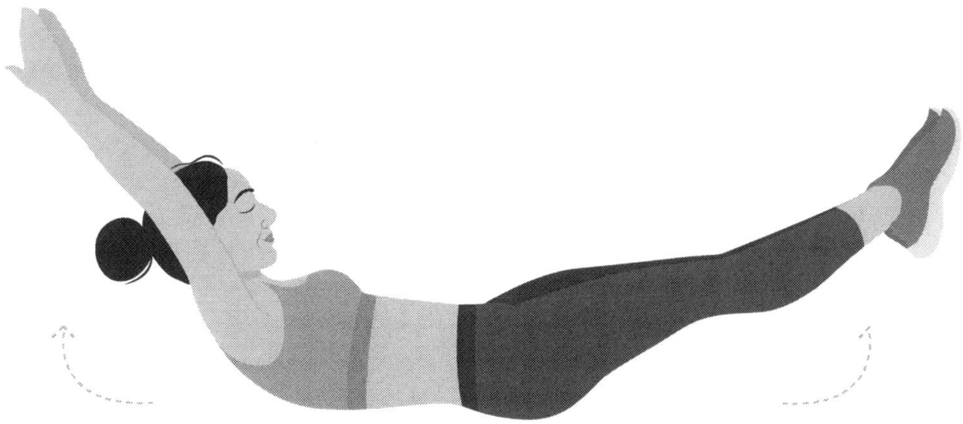

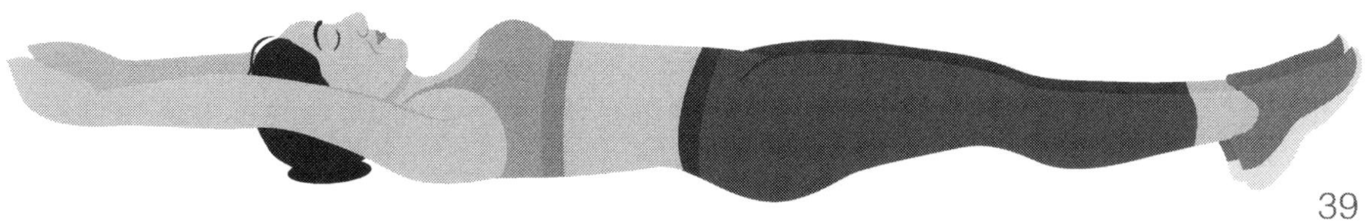

Long Lunge

The long lunge is a quad-dominant exercise developing single-leg strength and stability. The long lunge targets your quadriceps, thighs, hips, and glutes.

Instructions:

1. Begin standing tall with your feet shoulder-width apart.
2. Take a long step forward with your right foot while keeping your left foot planted.
3. Bend your right leg until it creates a 90-degree angle at the knee.
4. Ensure your shoulders are relaxed and your core is engaged.
5. Keeping the weight in your front heel, push the floor away to come back to your starting position.
6. Repeat the exercise on your opposite leg.

Tip: Keep your pelvis neutral, your chest high, and your back straight.

Easier Option: Feel free to cut back on the range of motion and stay above a 90-degree angle.

Harder Option: Hold weights at your side or wear a weighted backpack.

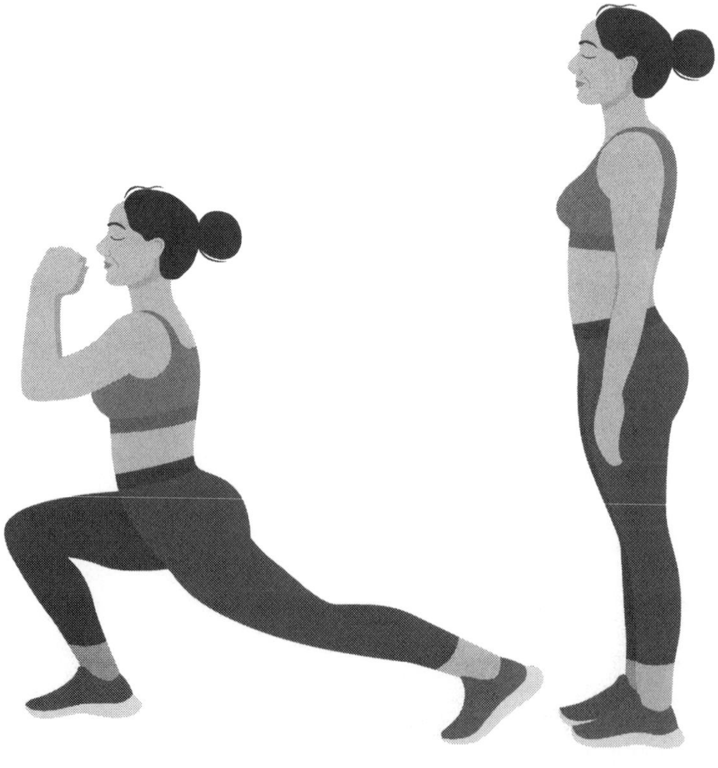

Hammer Curl

The hammer curl is a variation of the traditional bicep curl. However, your wrist remains in a fixed position to target additional muscles in your upper and lower arms.

Instructions:

1. Stand tall with your feet hip-width apart.
2. Hold a weight in each hand with your arms fully extended at your side.
3. Embrace your core and buttock.
4. Keep your palms facing your body and wrists held tight.
5. Bend at the elbow to bring the weight up to your shoulder.
6. Hold for a second before slowly lowering the weight back down.
7. Ensure your elbows remain pinned to your side.

Tip: Keep your wrists tight to work the smaller muscles in your hands. Don't let your wrists flop.

Easier Option: Perform the exercise without weights.

Harder Option: Lower the weight for a count of three seconds.

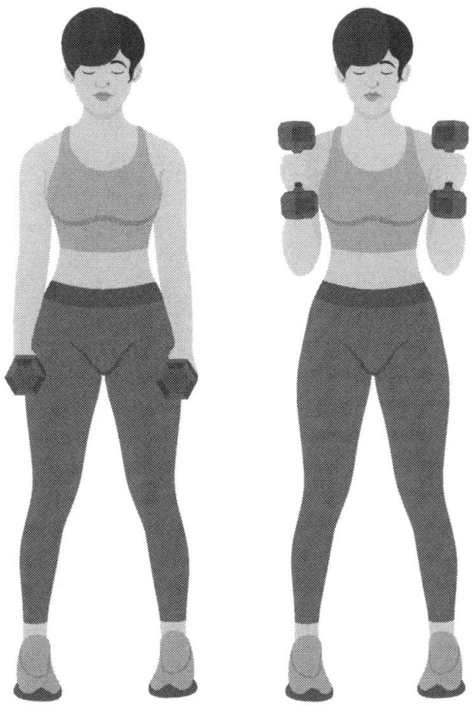

Calf Raises

Calf raises to build strength in the lower legs. Lower leg strength is vital for protecting your ankles from injury.

Instructions:

1. Stand tall with your feet just inside shoulder-width.
2. Point your toes forward.
3. Hold a weight in each hand.
4. Squeeze your shoulder blades together.
5. Push through the balls of the feet, raising your heels above your toes.
6. Hold for two seconds before slowly lowering.
7. Repeat this movement.

Tip: Place your toes on an elevated surface such as a book to increase the range of motion.

Easier Option: Perform the exercise without weights.

Harder Option: Do not let your feet touch the floor between reps. Keep tension in your lower leg by pausing half an inch from the floor.

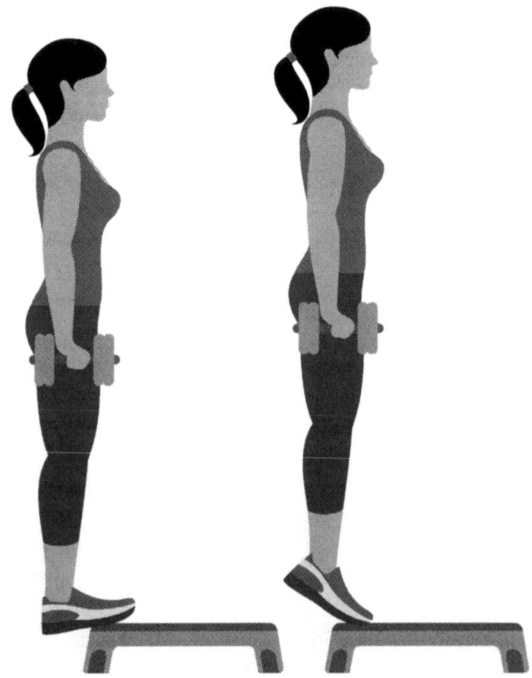

Boat

The boat pose develops core strength and stability in the back and abdomen. Specifically, it strengthens the abdominals, hip flexors, and spine.

Instructions:

1. Start with a sitting position with your knees bent and your feet flat on the floor.
2. Place your hands next to your hips.
3. Keeping your back straight, lean your torso back while lifting your feet off the floor.
4. Extend your legs and push your chest up.
5. Extend your arms forwards off the floor while maintaining a tight core.
6. Your body should now be in a V-shape.
7. Hold this position.

Tip: Spread your shoulder blades apart.

Easier Option: Bend your knees and keep your hands on the floor.

Harder Option: Lower your feet to an inch off the floor, then raise them back up to work the lower abdomen harder.

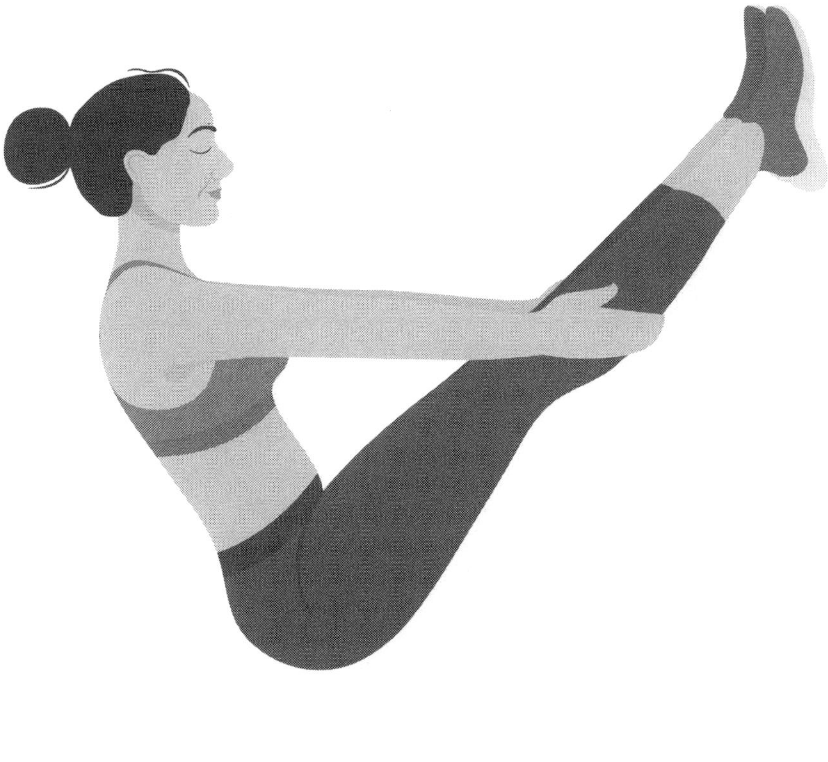

Plié Squat

The plié squat strengthens the quads, hamstrings, glutes, and calves while increasing the range of motion in your hips.

Instructions:

1. Stand with your feet outside shoulder-width apart.
2. Rotate your feet out to a 45-degree angle.
3. Put your hands on your hips.
4. Push your hips back and bend the knees until your buttock is just above knee height.
5. Drive through your mid-foot to return to standing.
6. During extension, push your knees out.

Tip: Keep your chest up.

Easier Option: Perform a wide squat.

Harder Option: Place a resistance band just above your knees.

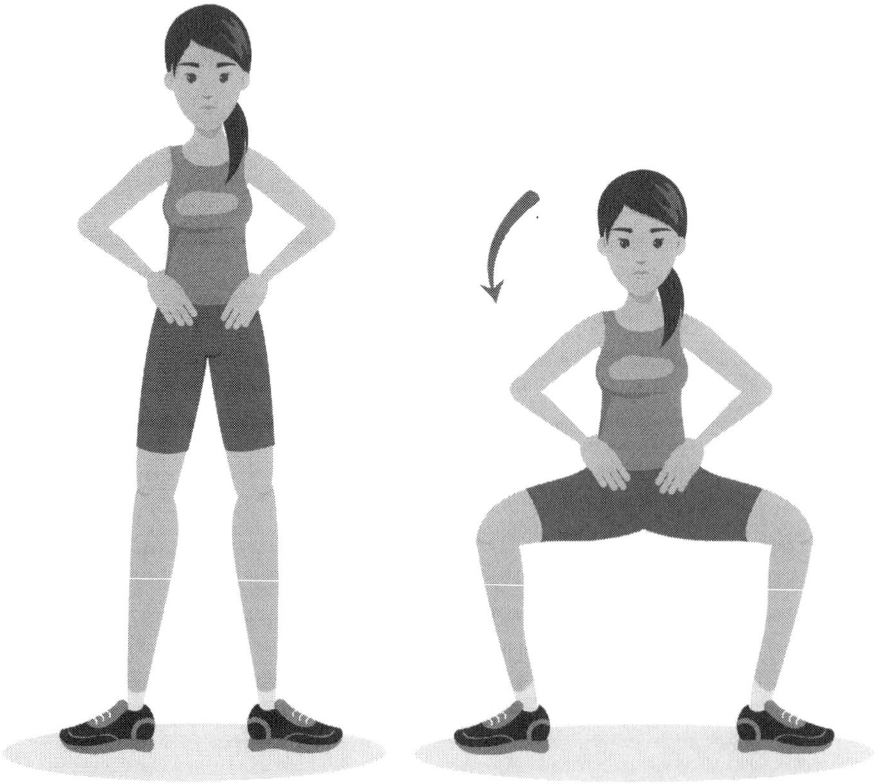

Split Stance Row

The split stance position improves your core and leg stability and strength. The rowing portion of the exercise works your shoulders, back, biceps, and triceps.

Instructions:

1. Stand tall with your feet shoulder-width apart and a weight in your right hand.
2. Step your left leg in front of you and your right leg behind - this is your split stance position.
3. Bend your left knee slightly, then lean your torso until it's close to parallel to the floor.
4. Engage your core and buttocks.
5. Bend your right elbow to pull the weight to your chest.
6. Pause for one second, then slowly lower to full extension.
7. Perform half the repetitions on your right side and the other half on your left.

Tip: Place your left hand on your left thigh for stability.

Easier Option: Perform the exercise without weights.

Harder Option: Pause for four seconds at the top of the movement.

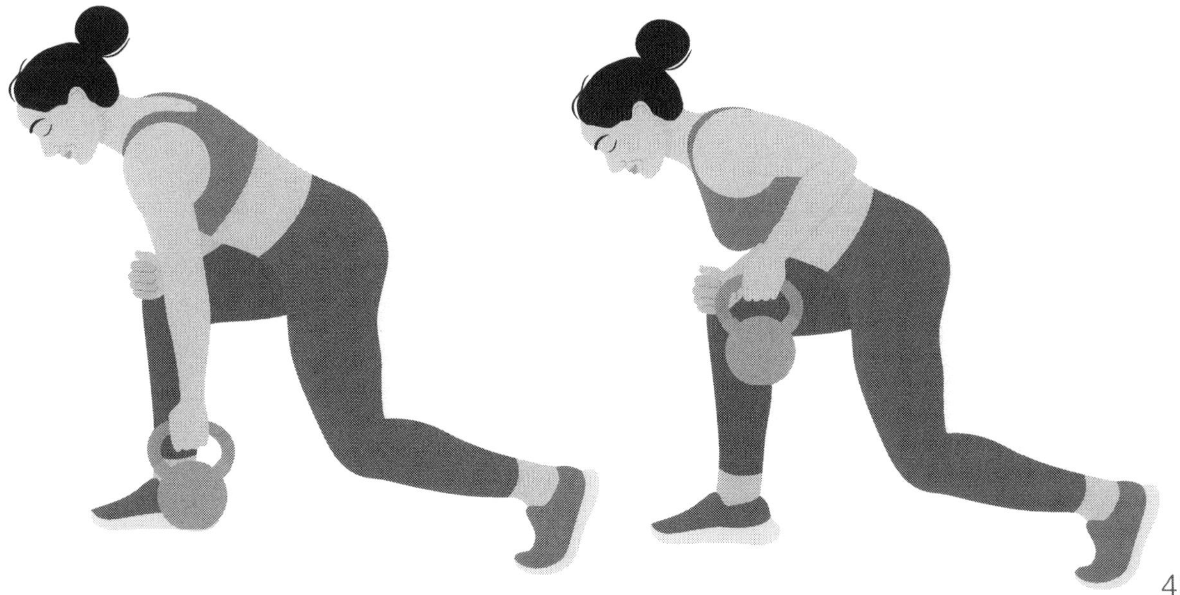

Donkey Kicks

Donkey kicks work your core and glute muscles to build strength and stability.

Instructions:

1. Start on your hand and knees.
2. Your hands should be directly under your shoulders and your knees under your hips.
3. Keep your back flat, core engaged, and glutes tensed.
4. Keeping your leg bent, raise your right leg until your thigh is in line with your torso.
5. Pause for one second before lowering to the starting position.
6. Repeat the movement on your left leg.

Tip: Keep your hips squared. Avoid any torso rotation.

Easier Option: Reduce the range of motion.

Harder Option: Place a resistance band above your knees.

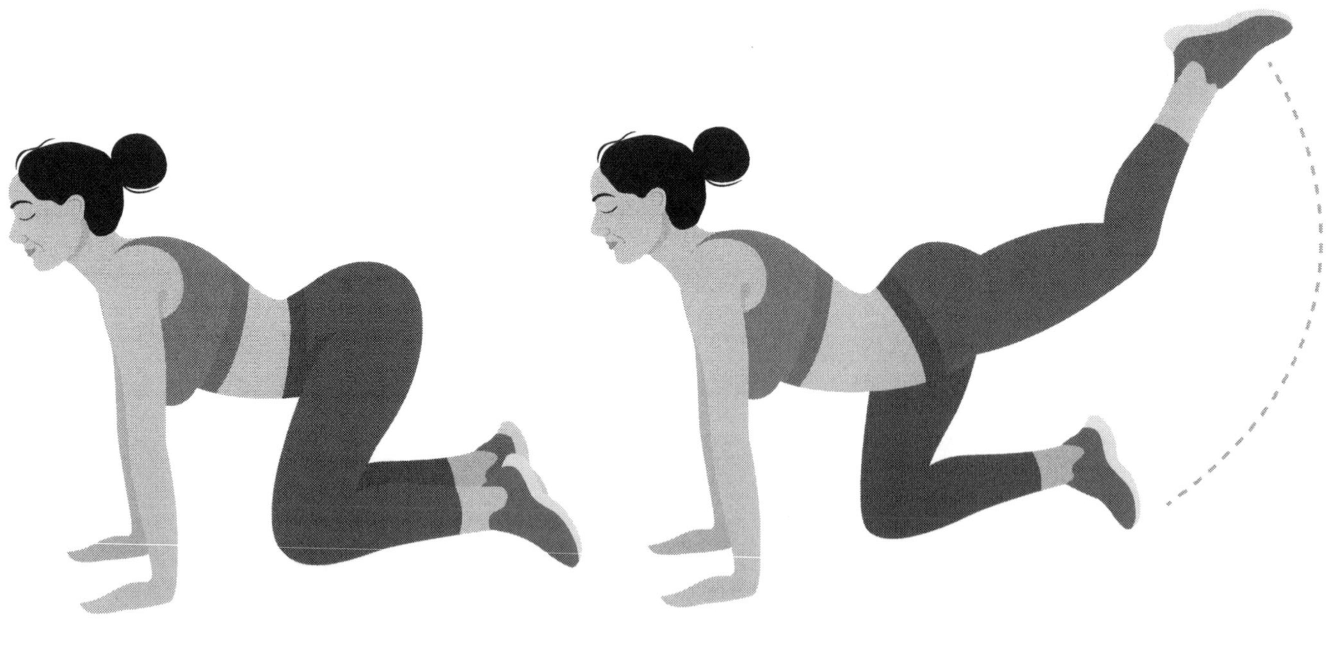

Leg Raises

Leg raises build your core strength and stability. Leg raises focus on the lower part of your abdominals, which can be difficult to target.

Instructions:

1. Begin lying on the floor with your legs extended and arms at your side.
2. Push your shoulders, upper back, and lower back into the floor while squeezing your core.
3. Squeeze your ankles together.
4. Lift your feet off the floor to a 90-degree angle.
5. Hold for a second before slowly lowering.

Tip: Control the movement, don't rely on momentum.

Easier Option: Bend your legs to a 90-degree angle.

Harder Option: Do not lower your legs to the floor. Pause an inch from the floor before performing the next repetition.

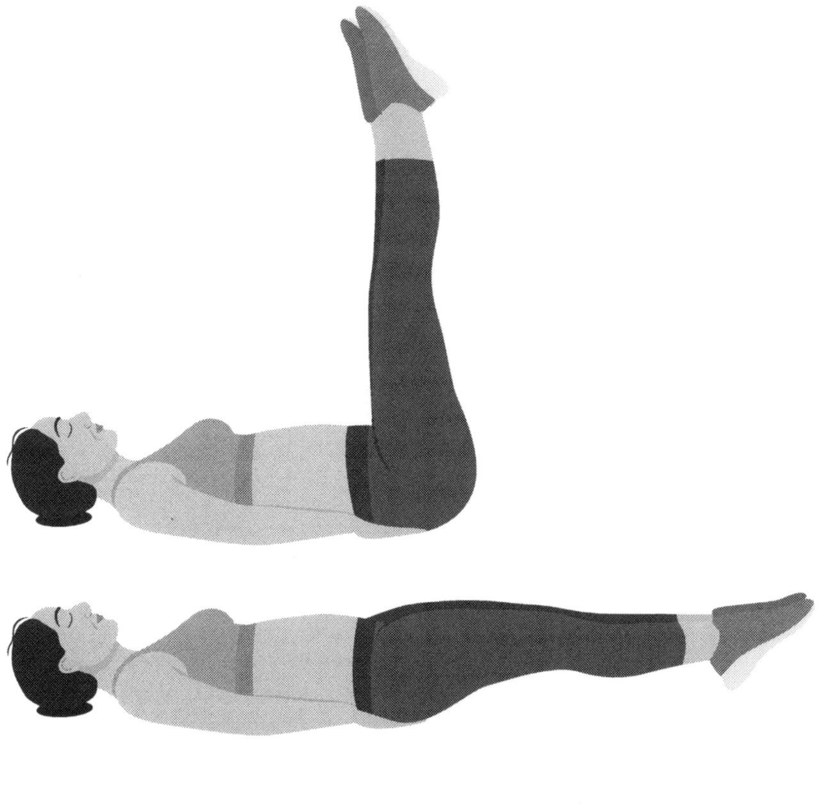

Single-Leg Box Squat

Single leg box squats are similar to bench squats, but focus on single-limb movement. Single limb movements help eliminate any muscle imbalances. The single-leg box squat develops strength in your glutes, hamstrings, and quads. This is a great crossover to real-life movements such as standing up out of a chair. If you don't have a box, use a raised surface of similar height, such as a chair, bench, or low wall.

Instructions:

1. To perform the single-leg box squat, stand with feet shoulder-width apart.
2. Squeeze your shoulder blades, core, and buttock.
3. Lift your right leg off the floor an inch or two.
4. Send your hips back and bend your left knee until you are sitting on the bench.
5. After a brief pause, drive your hips up to return to standing while keeping your core tight and back neutral.
6. Perform half the repetitions on your left leg and half on your right.

Tip: It's important to pause in the box. This exercise aims to eliminate any rebound movement.

Easier Option: Perform regular bench squats.

Harder Option: Hold a weight at chest height.

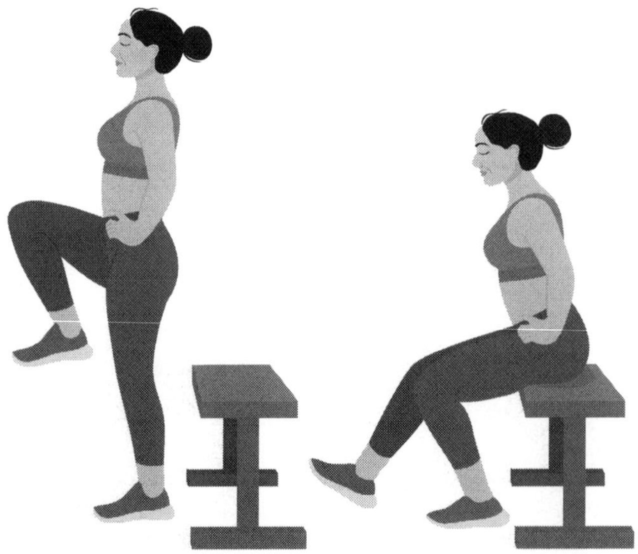

Shoulder Press

The shoulder press strengthens your shoulders and upper back. It's an excellent crossover for overhead press movement, such as putting your bag into overhead storage.

Instructions:

1. Stand tall with your feet hip-width apart with a weight in each hand.
2. Bend the elbows to bring the weights to your shoulders; this is your starting position.
3. Pull your shoulder back, engage your core, and squeeze your buttock.
4. Push the weights towards the sky until they reach full extension.
5. Pause for one second, then lower the weights back to the starting position.

Tip: Push your head forward during extension.

Easier Option: Perform the exercise without weights.

Harder Option: Perform the exercise on the floor with your legs extended and your torso upright.

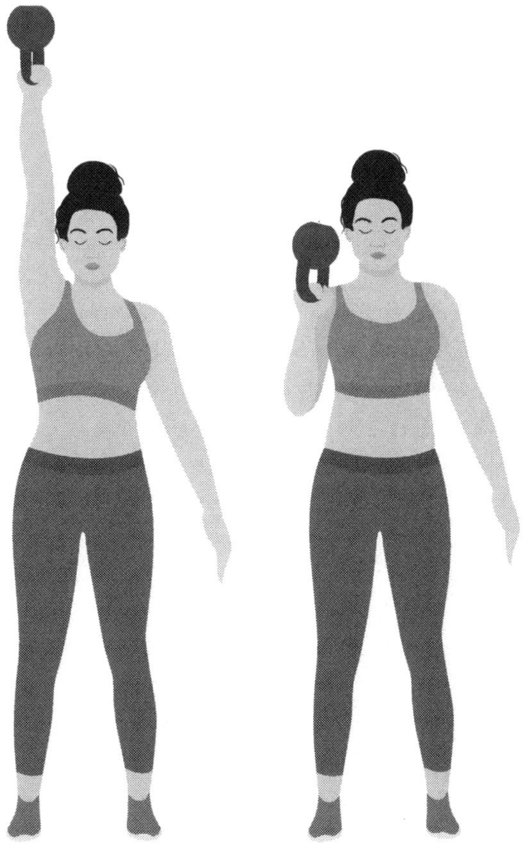

Reverse Lunges

Reverse lunges are a core, glute, and hamstring-focused exercise. Unlike regular lunges, we will be stepping back with our legs to initiate the movement rather than stepping forward. This places less stress on your joints and gives you more stability in your front leg. Therefore, it's a great exercise for those with knee problems, balance issues, or restricted hip mobility.

Instructions:

1. Begin standing with your feet hip-width apart.
2. Take a long step back with your right leg and bend your left knee until it reaches a 90-degree angle.
3. Keep your core and buttocks tight.
4. Drive through the mid-foot of your left leg to return to standing.
5. During the drive-up, push your left knee out to the side.
6. Repeat on the opposite side.

Tip: Focus on a specific place on the wall throughout the exercise to help with your balance.

Easier Option: Reduce the range of motion by staying above a 90-degree angle.

Harder Option: Hold a weight in each hand.

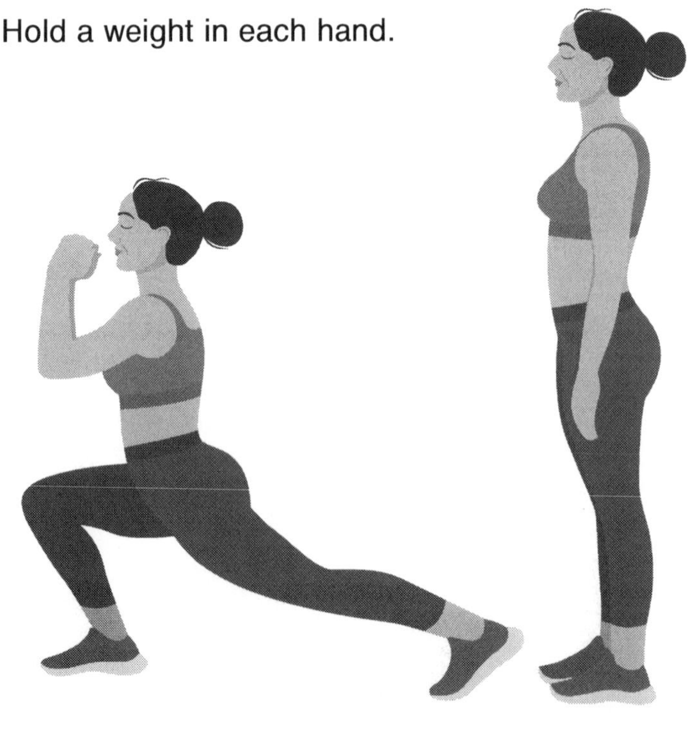

Sphinx

The sphinx strengthens your spine and glutes while stretching the chest, shoulders, and abdominals.

Instructions:

1. Begin lying on the floor face down.
2. Place your elbows under your shoulders and place your feet hip-width apart.
3. Push your feet and quads into the floor.
4. Push through your elbows to raise your chest and head.
5. Keep your hips on the floor and pull your shoulder blades together.
6. Hold this position.

Tip: Rotate your thighs inwards.

Easier Option: Place a rolled-up towel in a U-shape on the floor. Lie on the towel to support the lift.

Harder Option: Extend your arms fully.

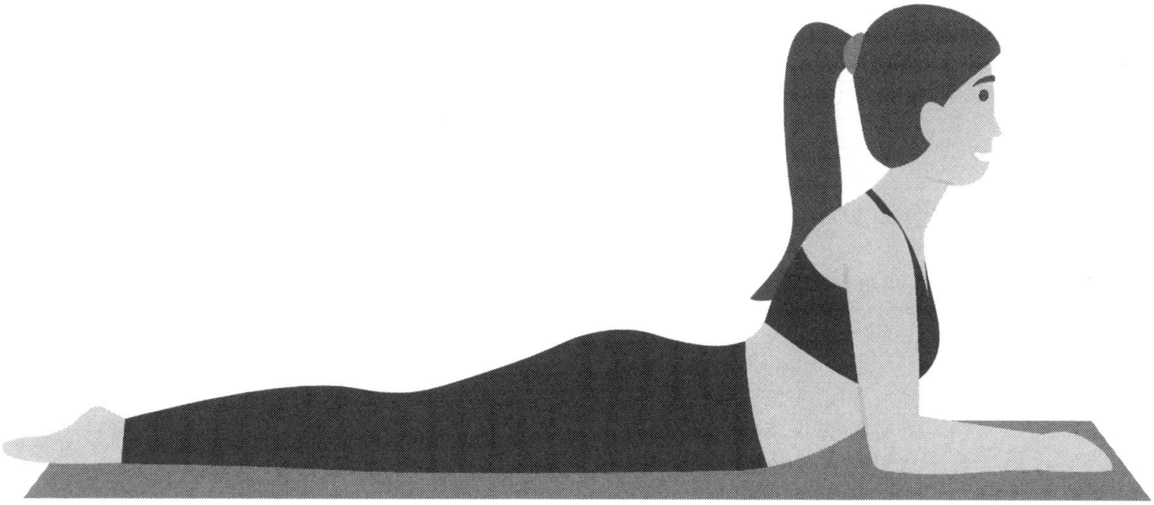

Single-Leg Raise

Single-leg raises are an advanced version of plank hip dips. They develop full-body strength and stability. The additional hip raise also puts more emphasis on the glutes.

Instructions:

1. Begin sitting on the floor with your legs extended and your torso upright.
2. Place your hands on the floor behind your shoulders.
3. Lean back so your arms take the weight of your body.
4. Bring your feet to your buttock while remaining flat on the floor.
5. Push through your feet and palms to lift your hips slightly off the floor.
6. From here, fully extend your left leg towards the sky.
7. Lift your hip and extend your arms.
8. Pause for one second, then lower back to the floor.
9. Perform half the repetitions on your right leg and half on your left.

Tip: Push through your foot on the floor to assist the lift.

Easier Option: Keep both feet on the floor.

Harder Option: Place a resistance band just above your knees.

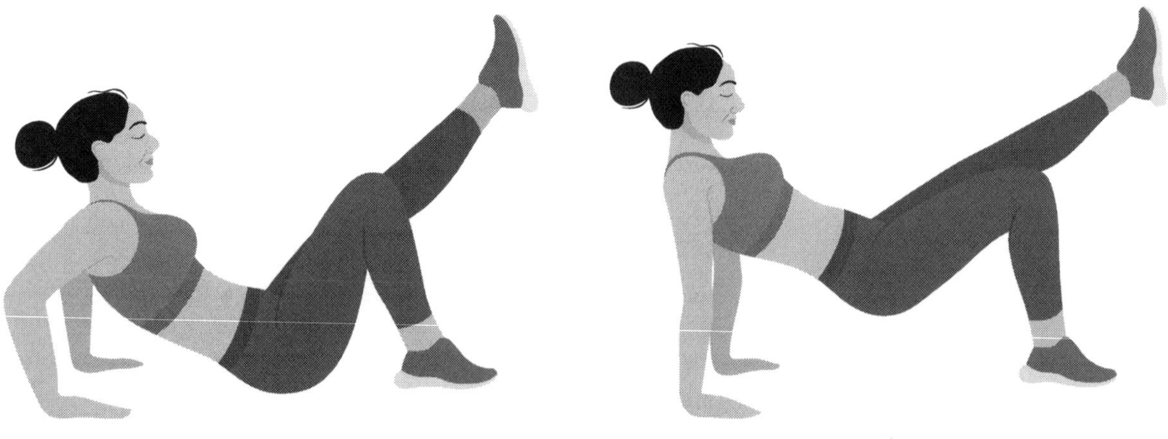

Lateral Raises

Lateral raises focus on building your shoulder strength, specifically your lateral shoulder strength. They also help strengthen the shoulder joint.

Instructions:

1. Stand tall with your feet hip-width apart and a weight in each hand at your sides.
2. Pull your shoulders back, squeeze your buttock, and engage your core.
3. Slightly bend your elbows, then lift the weight out to the side until your arms are parallel to the floor.
4. Pause for one second, then slowly lower back to the center.

Tip: Initiate the movement with your elbows.

Easier Option: Perform the exercise without the weights.

Harder Option: Reduce the range of motion to keep tension in the shoulders.

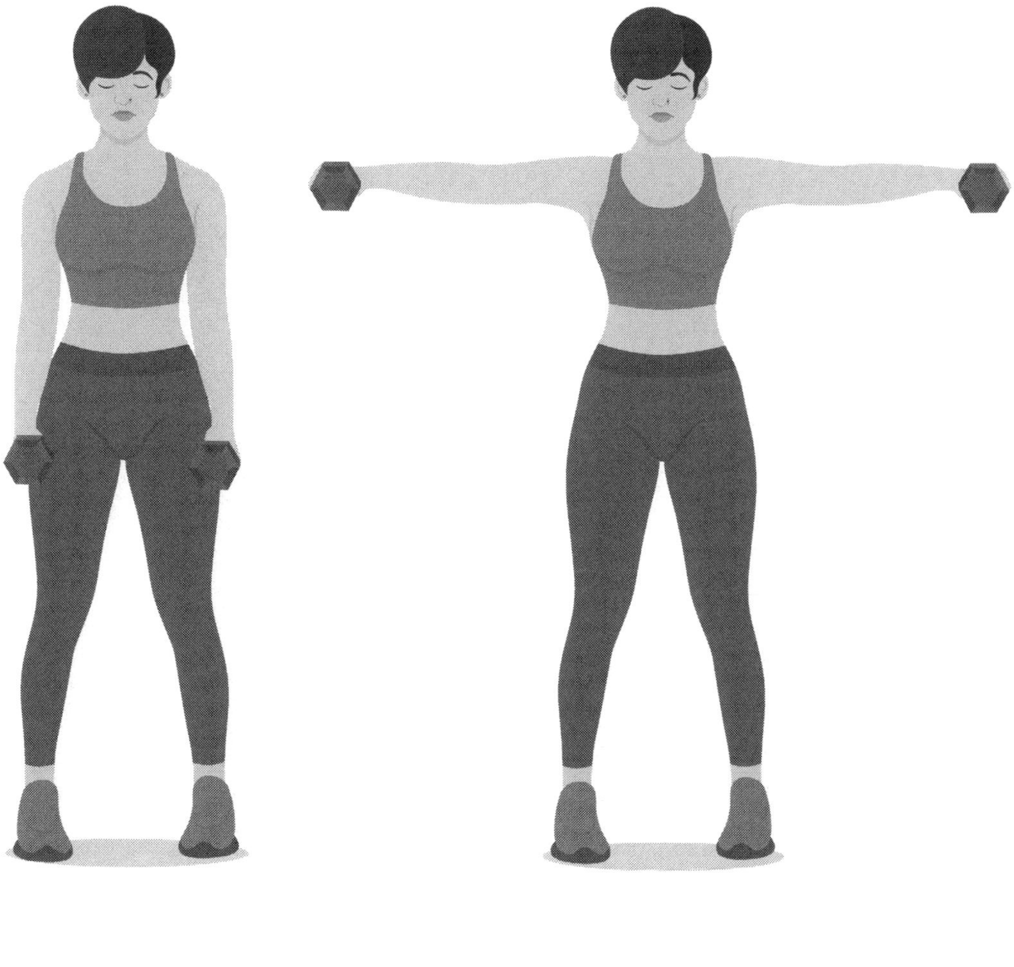

Side Lunges

Side lunges help improve your balance, strength, and stability. They work your inner and outer thighs, also known as your adductors and abductors. The sideways movement helps prepare your body for side-to-side movements such as shuffling during sports play.

Instructions:

1. Stand tall with your feet hip-width apart.
2. Take a wide step out to your right while bending your right knee as far as you can without rounding your back.
3. Keep both feet flat on the floor.
4. Push through your right foot to return to standing.
5. Repeat on your left side.

Tip: Point your knees in the same direction as your feet.

Easier Option: Step out to the side without bending your knee.

Harder Option: Hold a weight close to your chest.

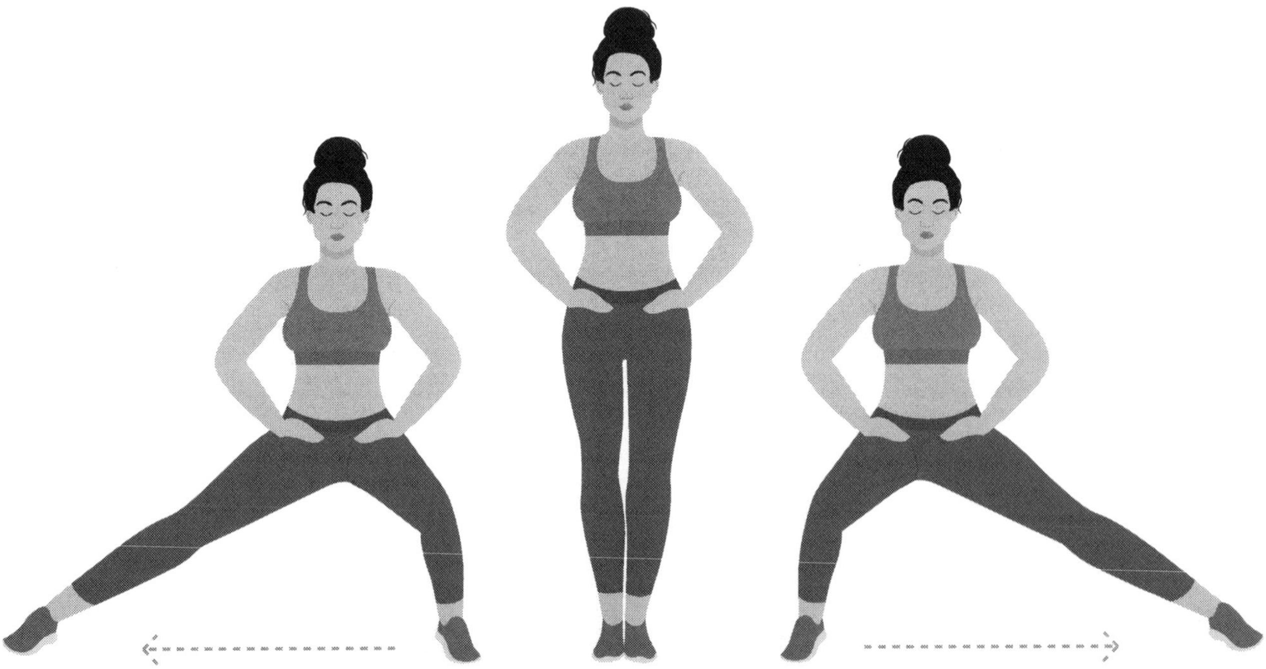

Cat-Cow

The cat-cow is a mobility exercise used to improve posture and balance. It also helps you relax while relieving stress.

Instructions:

1. Start on your hands and knees with your hips over your knees and shoulders over your hands.
2. From here, lower your chest without bending your arms.
3. Then, bring your upper back up towards the ceiling, rounding your shoulders.

Tip: Imagine a piece of string is attached to your chest, and someone is pulling it towards the floor and ceiling.

Easier Option: Perform the movement in a chair.

Harder Option: Work through the two positions in one fluid movement.

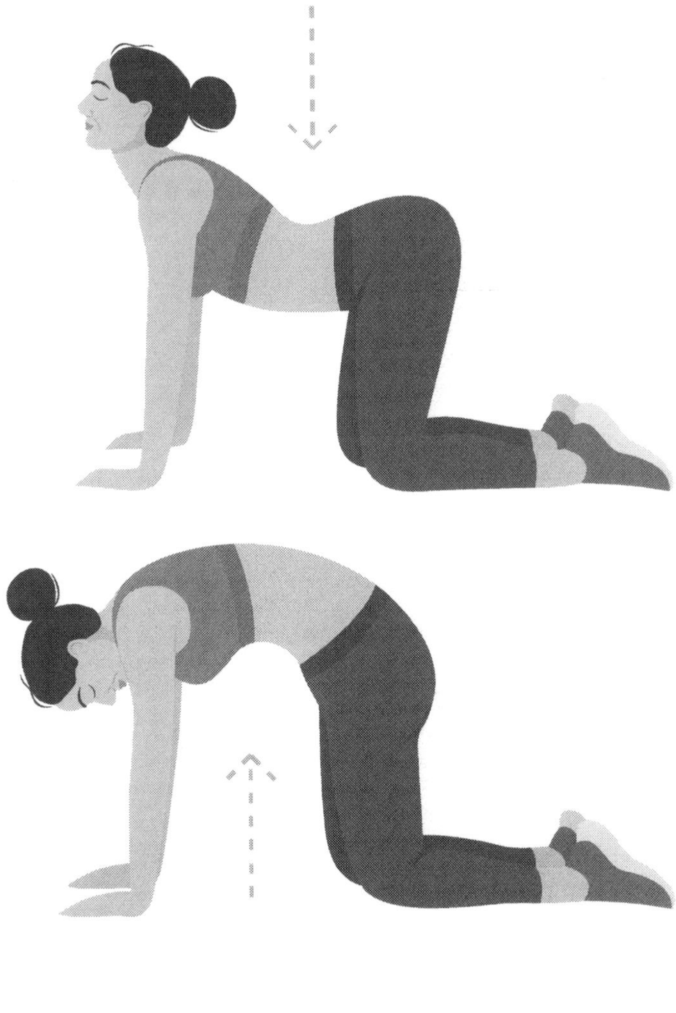

Knee to Elbow Extension

Knee to elbow extensions are similar to mountain climbers but focus more on the glutes. They also work your shoulders, hamstrings, quads, triceps, and core.

Instructions:

1. Begin in a press-up position with your arms and legs fully extended.
2. Your weight should be spread between your hands and feet.
3. Keep your shoulders, hips, and feet remain aligned throughout the move ment, as well as keeping your core engaged.
4. Bring your right knee towards your right elbow.
5. Drive your right foot back and raise your foot to the sky.
6. Pause for a second before returning to the starting position.
7. Repeat the movement on your left leg.

Tip: Lift your leg until you feel your glute fully contract.

Easier Option: Only perform the leg lift. Do not bring your knee to your elbow.

Harder Option: Place a resistance band just above your knees.

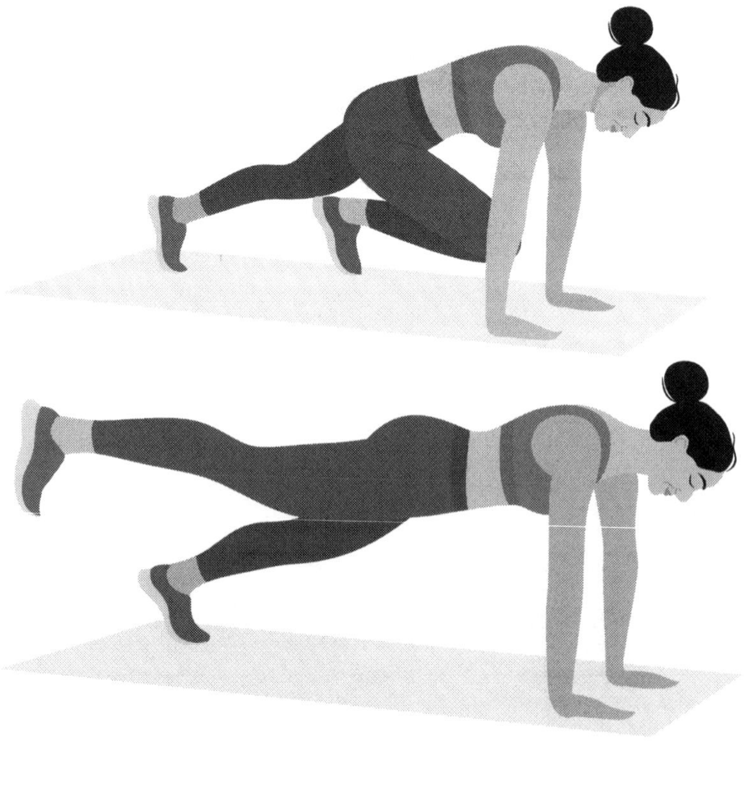

Shrugs

Shrugs build strength in your shoulders, neck, and upper back. They also help reduce neck and shoulder strain, as well as improve posture.

Instructions:

1. Stand tall with your feet hip-width apart.
2. Hold a weight in each hand at your sides.
3. Rotate your palms into your body.
4. Squeeze your core and buttock and draw your shoulder blades back.
5. Keeping your arms straight, lift your shoulders as high as possible.
6. Pause for one second before lowering to the starting position.

Tip: Imagine you are trying to touch your ears with your shoulders.

Easier Option: Perform the exercise without weights.

Harder Option: Perform the exercise with a barbell.

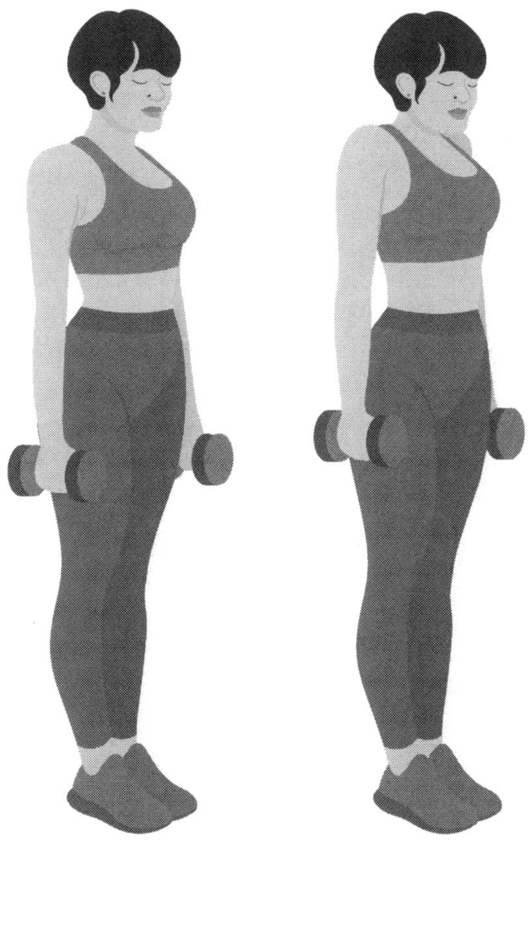

Wide Squat

Wide squats require more hip extension than regular air squats. Thus, it places more emphasis on hip strength. However, just like normal air squats, wide squats work your glutes, quads, hamstrings, calves, and core.

Instructions:

1. To perform the wide squat, stand with your feet outside shoulder-width apart.
2. Push your hips back and bend the knees until your buttock is just above knee height.
3. Drive through your mid-foot to return to standing.
4. During extension, push your knees out.

Tip: Initiate the movement from your hips, not your knees.

Easier Option: Bring your feet closer together to perform a regular air squat.

Harder Option: Hold a weight at chest height, or wear a weighted backpack.

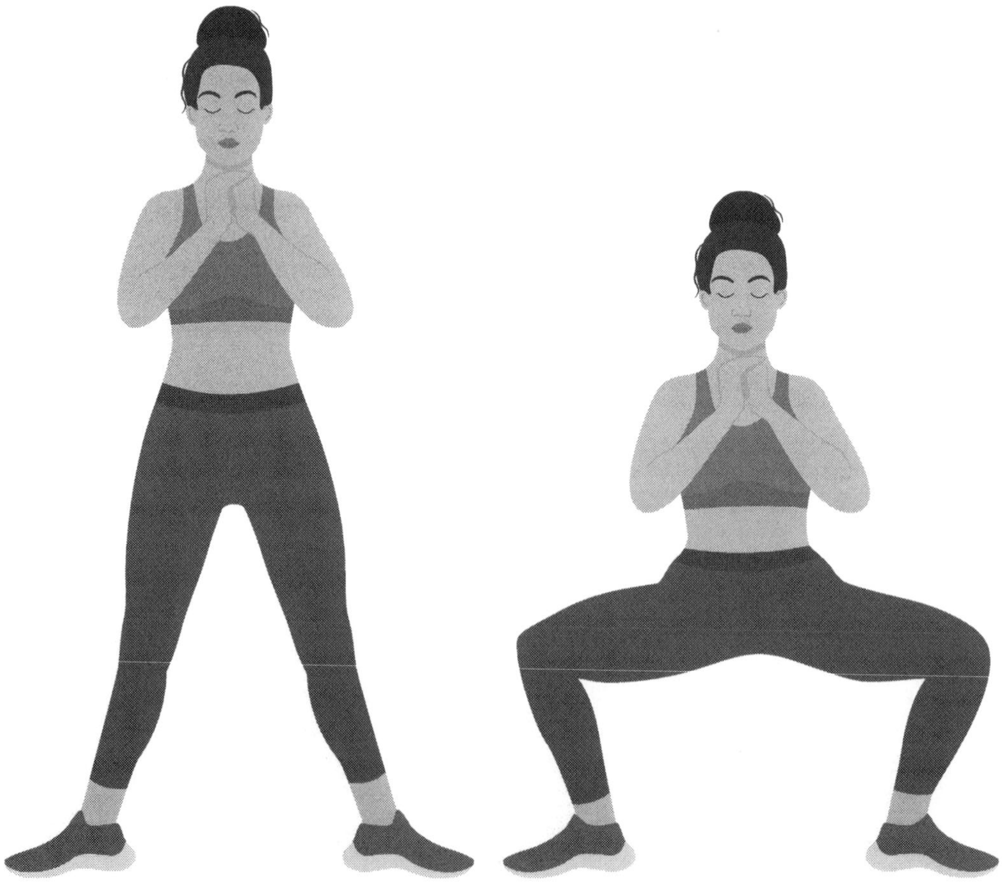

Cobra

The cobra improves your posture and alleviates back pain by strengthening the shoulders, arms, and back muscles.

Instructions:

1. Begin lying on the floor face down.
2. Place your hands by your ribs and place your feet hip-width apart.
3. Push your feet and quads into the floor.
4. Push through your palms to raise your chest and head.
5. Keep your hips on the floor and pull your shoulder blades together.
6. Hold this position.

Tip: Keep a slight bend in your arms.

Easier Option: Place your forearms on the floor and don't fully extend your arms.

Harder Option: Rest your feet on a book or block to extend the stretch.

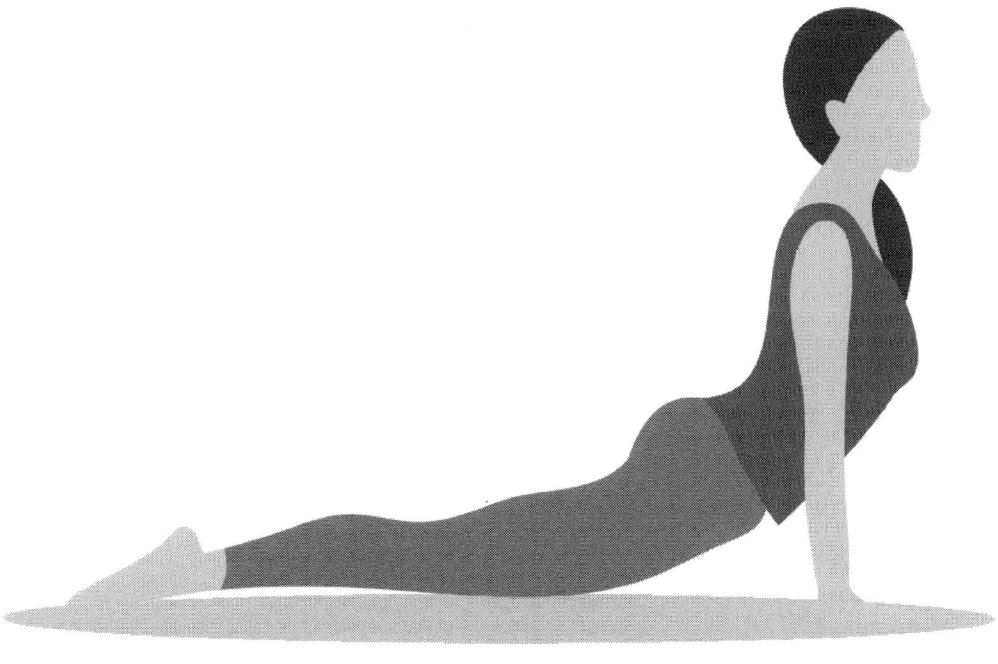

Chapter 2: **Stretching Exercise**

Think about that slow stretch of the body you do right after you get up in the morning. How good does that feel? Stretching is a great way to warm up the muscles, get rid of stiffness, improve circulation, and release endorphins that reduce pain and boost pleasure. We do it naturally and even involuntarily since we were babies. In fact, humans are not the only animals who love a good stretch. If you have a cat or a dog, you have probably seen them stretching after a good nap, or even when they are feeling bored after sitting somewhere for too long. Stretching is nature's reset button. It awakens your body and relaxes tight and stiff muscles. Especially as you age, it is important to include stretching in your day-to-day life since it will reduce pains and help you stay flexible and active.

What Happens When You Stretch?

Stretching involves deliberately straightening or extending your body parts to their full length or as much as you are able to extend them. You have over 600 muscles in your body; they are made of fibrous elastic tissue. Muscle tissue contains muscle fibers, each consisting of a single muscle cell.

These fibers can contract, relax, and elongate. When you stretch, your muscle fiber is pulled to its full length. This helps your muscle to realign any disorganized fibers in the direction of any tension or stiffness you have. This realignment is what helps nurse any scarred tissue back to health when you recover from a muscle injury. It also helps heal and recover the muscles that get fatigued often as you age.

When you stretch your muscles, depending on their location in your body, some of their fibers lengthen, and some of them remain at rest. The length of your muscle depends upon the number of stretched fibers at any given time. As you learn about the importance of stretching, it is also important to understand the way our brain and the neural components adapt to stretching. When your muscles stretch, the nerve control points located among the muscle groups called muscle spindles also stretch. The function of these muscle spindles is to protect the body from injury and maintain the tone of the muscle. They record the way the length of the muscle changes due to stretching and signals the brain, triggering the stretch reflex, which contracts the muscle. When you stretch suddenly, these muscle contractions will be strong and uncomfortable. This is why you have to ease into your stretching.

Benefits of Stretching After 40

It is natural to lose some of the functionality you enjoyed in your bright-eyed and bushy-tailed younger years once you pass the age of 40. As a part of the aging process, your muscles become less elastic, and you cannot lengthen them as you used to. However, the ability of your muscles to be trained does not stop with age. If you put some time every day into helping them, be more flexible, especially with resistance training preceded and followed by a full-body stretching session, you can prolong the time your muscles stay young and healthy. In fact, stretching and strength training are proven to minimize your age-related muscle loss and bone-related disorders.

Reduces Your Risk of Injury

When your body is warmed up and flexible, it is less likely that you would get injured when you work out or do any type of excessive movement. Stretching helps increase your range of movement, and it also helps decrease any resistance your muscles have, making it easier for you to do more intense strength training exercises. When you stretch both sides of your body, you are also helping remedy any muscular imbalances you have, further reducing muscle cramps and similar painful contractions.

Makes Your Body More Flexible and Pliable

Aging often makes your joints and muscles stiff, which leads to less flexibility. Stretching is an effective way to improve it since it increases the length your muscle can lengthen, helping you move with ease. When you stretch, your muscles' temporality lengthens, and it automatically returns to their normal length. When you do not move your muscles much, they become more and more resistant to being stretched. Practicing stretching regularly keeps your muscles ready and improves their elasticity, which you can then use for more intense exercises such as strength training.

Help Reduce Stress

Relieving muscle tension directly impacts your mental state. Stretching, when done properly, is similar to a massage to your sore joints and muscles. A good stretching session often takes time, and it allows you to connect with your body and for your thoughts to slow down. As you relieve the stress that you are carrying on your muscles when you stretch, you are also entering a meditative state that relieves your mental stress as well. Reducing stress from both your body and mind helps you sleep better as well.

Reduces Age-Related Aches and Pains

Stretching increases the blood flow to your muscles and improves your circulation overall. This helps the muscles receive more oxygen and get rid of any metabolic waste products causing discomfort. It also releases endorphins, a chemical that is produced in your central nervous system that have great pain-relieving effects.

Improves Your Posture

You are putting your muscles to work when you stretch. You are lengthening them, strengthening them, and basically making them do their job that they do not get to do due to the inactive modern lifestyles that we live. As a result, you will use any tightness or awkward muscle tensions that lead to bad posture. Stretching pulls your spine into positions that help make better connections with your back, neck, and core muscles, giving you a better posture. With regular stretching, you will notice that you are able to sit up straight with comfort and stand tall with good posture and a straight back.

Safety Tips

If you are new to working out and conscious stretching that warms you up for the more intense exercises that come after, there are quite a few safety tips that you should know beforehand. If you stretch incorrectly, the chances are that it will do more harm than good.

Here are some tips for safe stretches:

You Need to Warm Up Before Stretching

Since stretching is considered a warm-up, many people tend to plunge right into stretching before a workout. However, stretching cold muscles can lead to painful strains. Before you start your stretching session, do some light walking, jogging, or using an elliptical bike at low intensity for about ten minutes to warm up your muscles. Just like taffy, warm muscles are easier to stretch!

Aiming for Pain Is Bad

One of the most harmful beliefs in the fitness community is that if you feel pain, then you are doing a good job. This is not true when it comes to stretching. Your aim should be to feel mild to moderate tension when you stretch. The moment you start feeling pain, hold the stretch. You can try to reset your position carefully and then try again if you wish, but do not try to push through the pain. Do not worry. With constant and consistent practice along with strength training, your flexibility will inevitably improve.

Symmetry Is Key

Our bodies naturally change as we age, and losing flexibility is often a part of it. When you are getting into strength training after the age of 40, it is always important to keep your expectations attainable. This applies to stretching as well. If you strive to be as flexible as a twenty-year-old ballet dancer when you stretch, it is likely that you will get hurt and discouraged soon. Your focus should be to attain equal flexibility on both sides of your body. When your flexibility is not equal, it can be a risk factor when you are strength training later on.

Avoid Bouncing

A common mistake that beginners tend to make when stretching is making bounce motions to extend the stretch. This can be harmful and lead to injuries. It's okay to make gentle movements such as yoga, which helps improve your balance, but avoid rigid and bouncy movements when you stretch. Take your time with the stretch and be smooth when you move while keeping a steady posture. Do not try to rush through your stretching session before the workout. In fact, the longer you take, the less pain and resistance you will feel when you do your strength training.

Remember to Breathe

Breathe. Inhale and exhale consciously and with purpose when you stretch. Deep breathing lowers stress and stabilizes your blood pressure, which is extremely important before you move on to more intense strength training workouts.

Upper Body Stretching

Your upper body includes your neck and collarbone area, shoulders and arms, the chest—including breasts in women, back, stomach, hips, and the general waist area. Warming up and stretching your upper body is crucial to avoid any injuries during or after your strength training, especially after 40. The following stretching exercises will help release any stress in your upper body, loosen your joints, and get your blood flowing to your muscles.

Shoulder Circles

This is an easy upper body stretch to get you warmed up. It helps relax and build muscle tone in your shoulder area, triceps, and biceps. You can do it either standing or sitting, and it is discreet enough to do even at your work.

How to:

- Stand or sit in a neutral position with your back straight.
- Pull your shoulders back and open up your chest; inhale deeply and exhale fully, let your body feel heavy and relaxed.
- Raise your shoulders and rotate them slowly forward. Do up to 10 reps, or until you feel a stretch in your triceps. Pause, relax for a moment.
- Repeat the exercise in reverse.

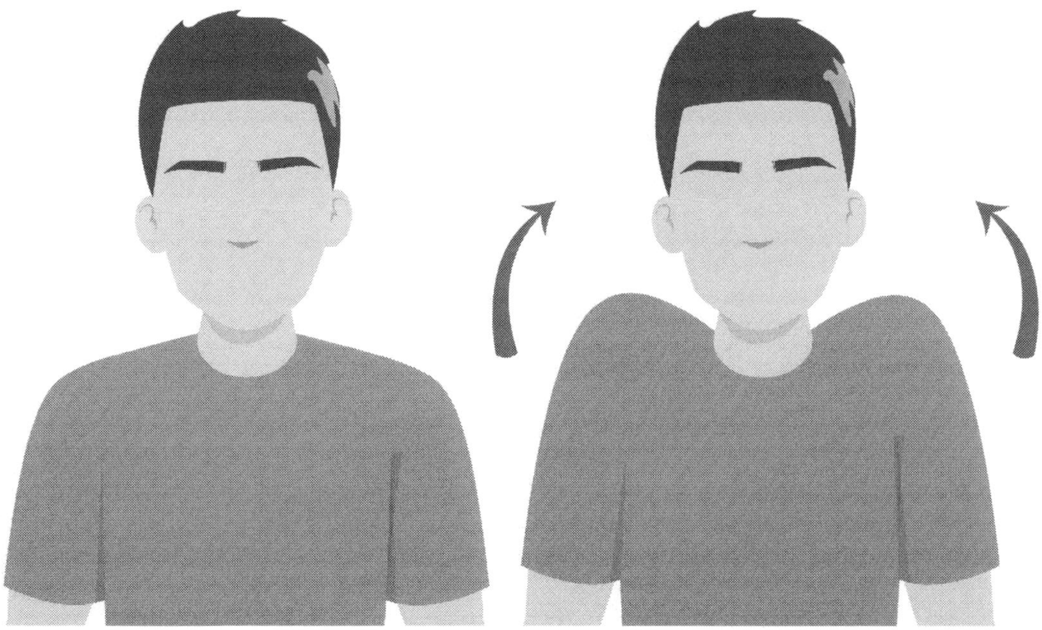

Cross-Body Shoulder Stretch

This is another upper-body stretch that warms up your shoulders, arms, and chest. While sitting or standing, you can do it, but make sure you keep your back and chin straight for better posture and results.

How to:

- Stand tall or sit with your back straight. Relax your body. Inhale and exhale.
- Bring one arm in front of you. Use the opposite hand to grab the elbow and pull it across your body towards your chest. Move the opposite hand from the elbow towards the shoulder and gently press until you feel the stretch in your shoulder.
- Keep your elbow slightly below your shoulder height and pause for 10–30 seconds.
- Repeat on the other side.

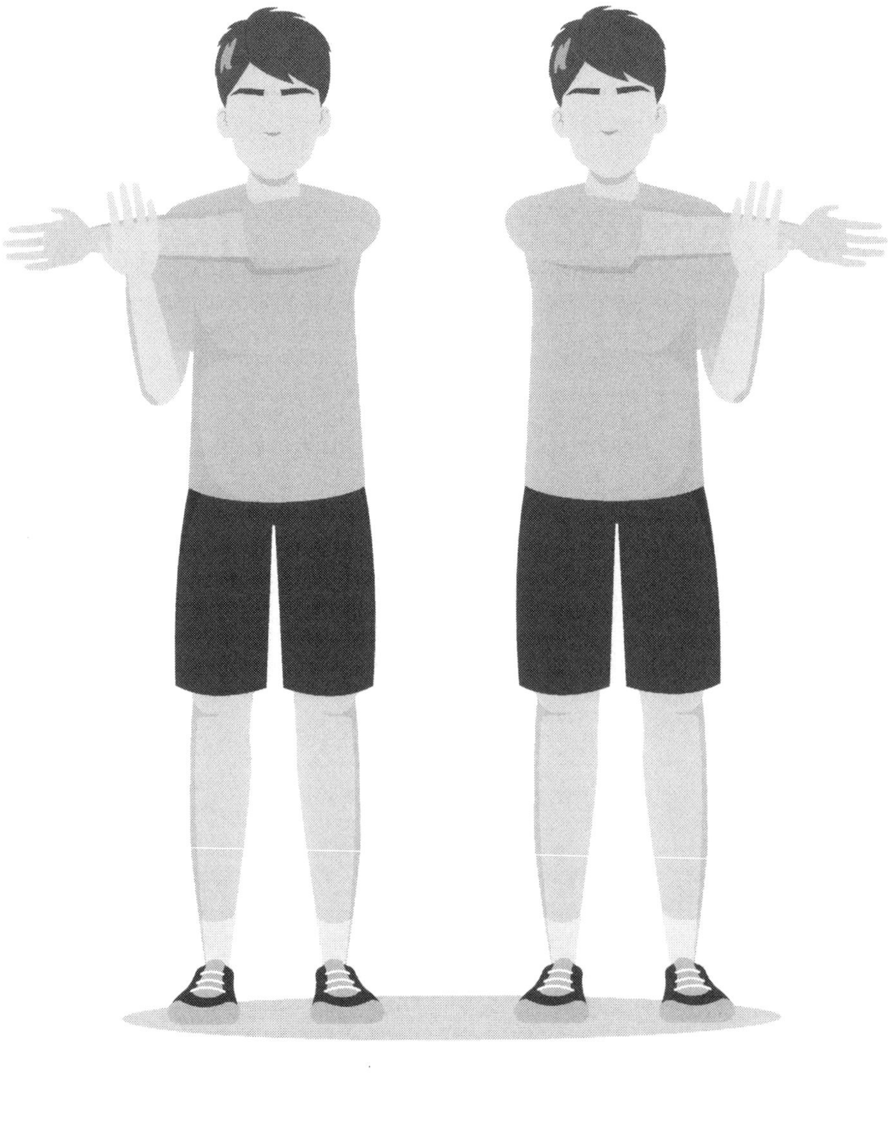

Lateral Raise and External Rotation

This exercise targets your entire chest area and is better done with a light pair of dumbbells. It is ideal before an upper-body strength training session.

How to:

- Stand tall and let your arms drop on either side of you. Take a deep breath and exhale slowly.
- Grab your light dumbbells and hold them at arm's length.
- Bend your elbows 90 degrees. Turn your palms towards each other, firmly holding dumbbells.
- Slowly raise your upper arms to the sides until they are at your chest height and parallel to the floor.
- Rotate your upper arms towards up and then back, so your forearms are pointed towards the ceiling. Pause.
- Reverse the movement and return to your starting position. Repeat.

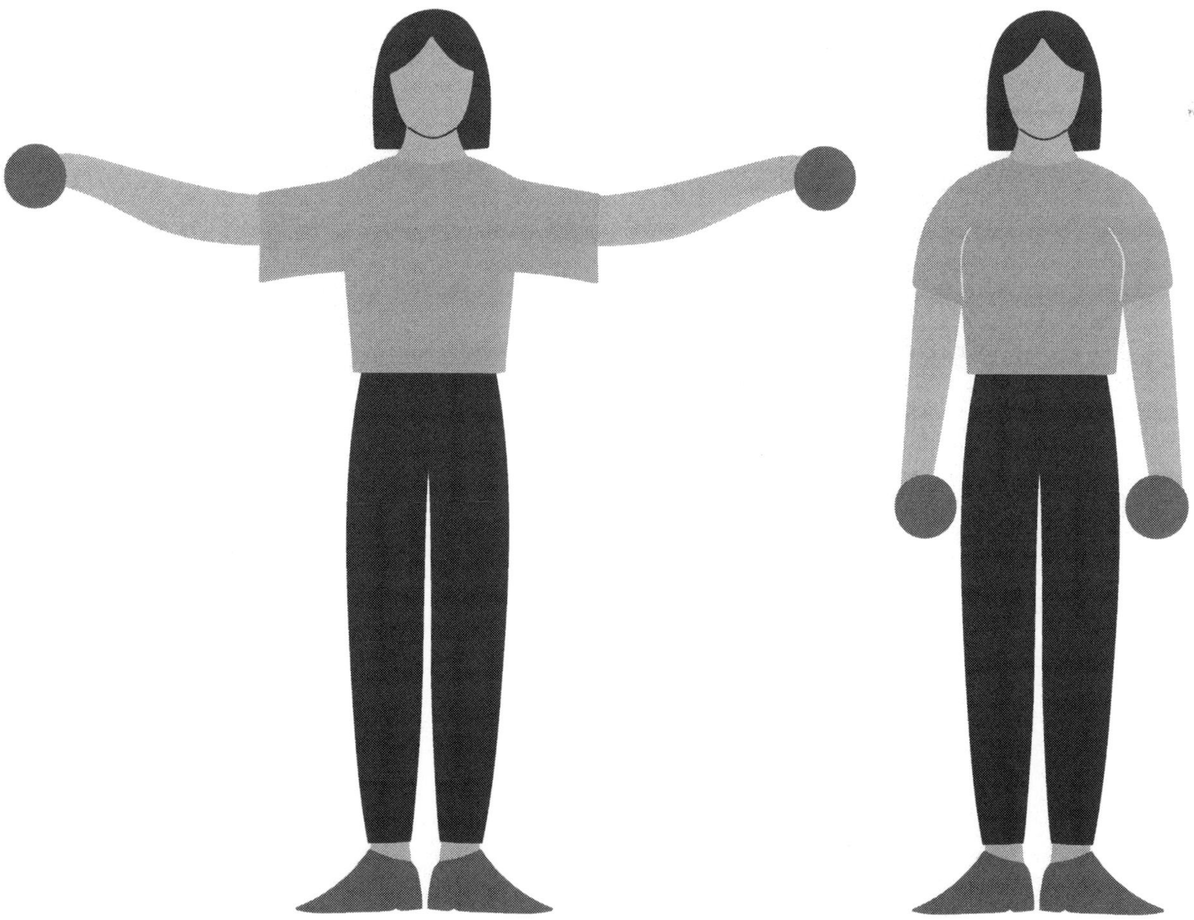

Lower Body Stretching

Your lower body is made of some of the biggest muscle groups in your body, including your hamstrings, quads, and the glutes on your back. Stretching your lower body helps you do the intense strength training exercises targeting that area, improving the flexibility of what is essentially your body's foundation. If you think of your body as a house, your lower body is the strong foundation that holds the rest of it. By warming up, you can avoid and reduce the pains and discomforts that may occur during strength training.

Calf Stretch

This is a classic exercise that targets your calf muscles. It does not require any equipment, and even beginners can do it easily and effectively. It is a great way to remove any tension in your lower body before you start your workout.

How to:

- Stand tall with your feet shoulder-width apart. Relax your body.
- Step the right foot forward and keep your left foot firmly on the ground.
- Bend your right forward until you feel the stretch on your calf muscles. Do not move your knee past your ankle. Hold for up to 30 minutes or as long as you can.
- Switch and repeat.

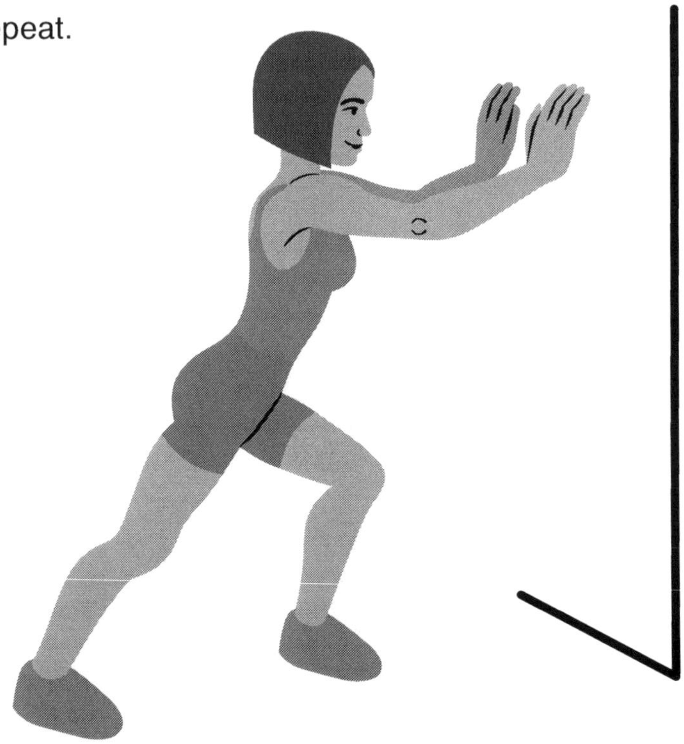

Full Body

A full-body stretch includes stretching and warming up all the main muscle groups in your body, including your chest, back, arms, abdominals, legs, and shoulders. Whether you engage in a more intense strength training session later or simply feel like relieving any stiffness in your body, a full-body stretch is infinitely beneficial. It helps you avoid injuries and may also help reduce the mobility issues that arise after the age of 40.

Child's Pose

Inspired by the Yoga pose "Balasana," Child's Pose is a great full-body stretch that uses the muscles of your lower back, inner thighs, and arms. It is an easy and comfortable pose that anyone can do regardless of their age. Apart from all the stretching benefits, Child's pose is great as a stress reliever and an easy remedy for back pain.

How to:

- Kneel on a mat with your thighs perpendicular to the floor, your shins parallel to the floor, and your head facing forward.
- Slowly put your feet together behind you, with your toes touching each other.
- Lower your hip backward as far as you can, and sit on your heels. Rest your belly on your thighs.
- Extend your arms in front of you and slowly rest your forehead on the floor.
- Fully give into the long stretch from top to bottom, and let your shoulders and back feel the stretch fully. Deepen the stretch as much as you can. Relax your body.
- Hold for up to 30 seconds, or for as long as you feel good.

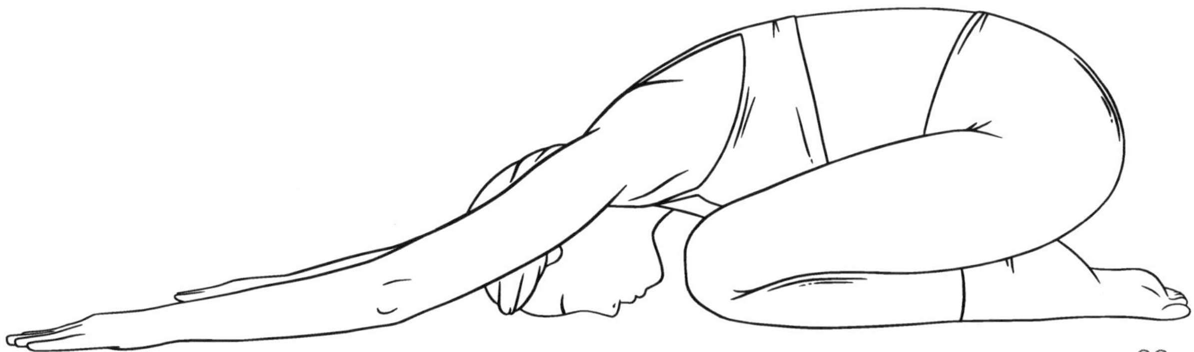

Glute Stretch

This stretching exercise targets your glutes and hips. You can do this both before and after your strength training to ease any aches and pains, removing any remaining tension on your back.

How to:

- Lie on your back and relax your body. Fill your lungs with a full inhale and ex hale fully.
- Bring your legs up until your toes point to the ceiling and bend your knees at 90 degrees.
- Use your hands to place your left ankle over your right knee.
- Hold your right leg firmly behind your knee and pull it towards your face. Feel the stretch on your glutes.
- Hold for 30 seconds. Switch legs and repeat.

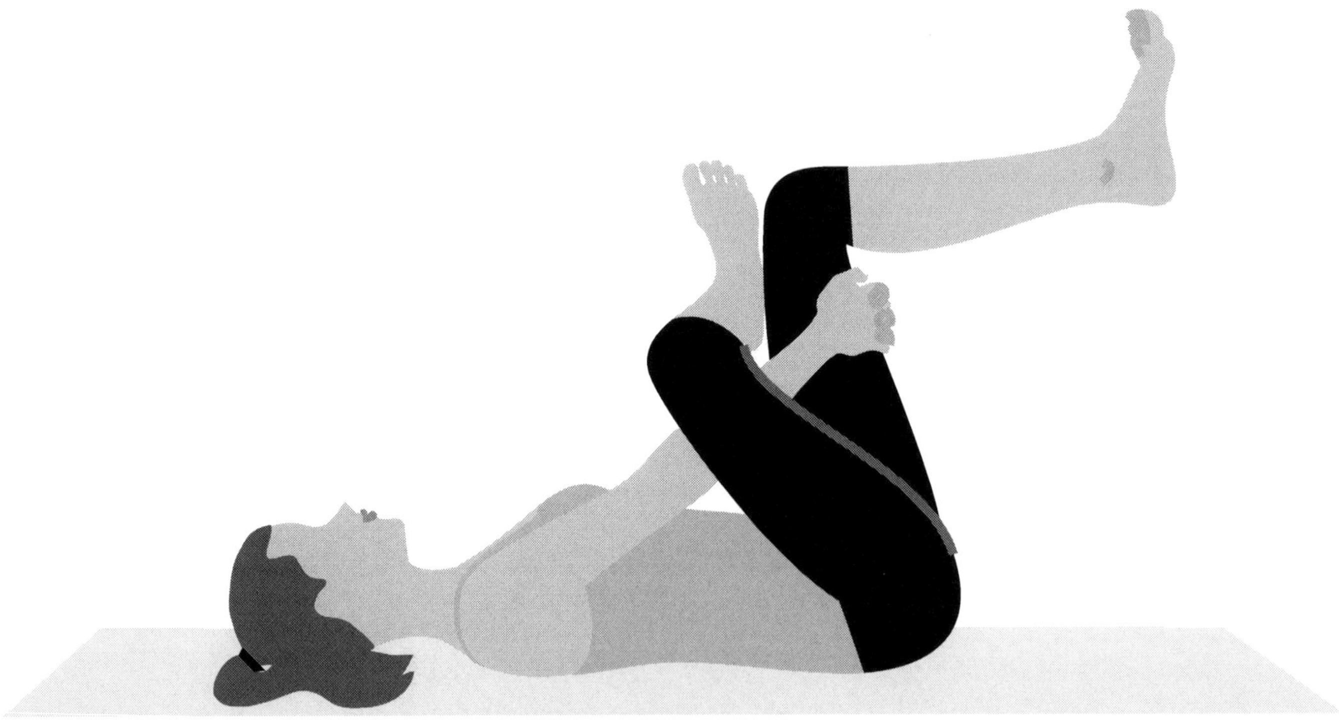

Downward Dog

While it may sound and appear complex, Downward Dog is one of the easiest fully body stretches that you can do, readying your body for strength training. Apart from building strength, this stretch also increases your flexibility and relieves back pain. Make sure you do some initial upper and lower body warm-up exercises before you attempt this full-body stretch.

How to:

- Get into a push-up position, with your legs together, and your hands kept firmly on the floor shoulder-width apart.
- Keep your body straight and your core fully engaged. In that position, slowly move your hips up, forming a V shape with your body, like a mountain. You can slightly bend your knees if you feel too much discomfort.
- Lower your head and place it between your shoulders while keeping your body steady. Feel your body stretch from your neck to your toes. Deepen your stretch by raising your heels.
- Hold the pose for 20–30 seconds. Return to your starting position.

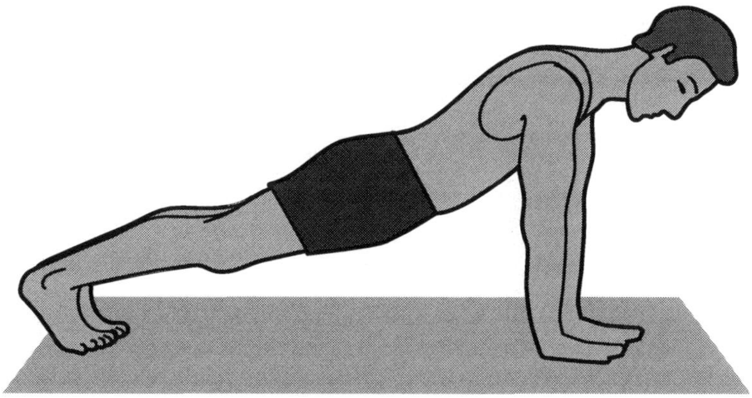

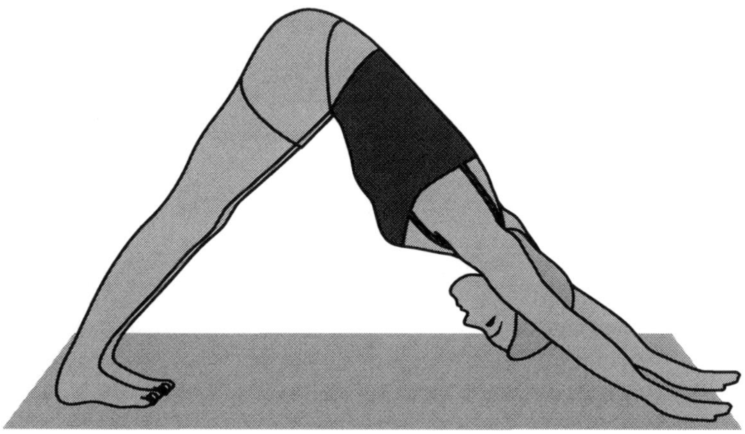

Chapter 3: **Yoga Exercises**

Chair Yoga

Chair yoga, which was first introduced to the fitness community as a modified form of Hatha Yoga for people with health issues and the elderly, has developed many new fans. With the amount of time people spend sitting at their offices or flying on long flights, there is a push to incorporate more activity and circulation into our everyday routines. Chair yoga can help our bodies by increasing flexibility, relieving cramps and stiffness, and promoting a positive mental attitude.

Chair yoga is a style of yoga that can be performed sitting or standing with the help of a chair. It is ideal for people who can't stand, don't have the agility to switch easily from standing to seated positions and vice versa, or just want a fast break from office work. Chair Yoga is also appropriate for someone immobile, has a physical disability, or has a mental disorder such as dementia or Alzheimer's. Research shows that chair yoga reduces pain, pain interference, and fatigue while also improving gait speed (Park et al., 2017).

Particulars

Difficulty Level: Easy

Equipment Needed: A chair.

Repetitions: Do ten of each variant.

Performing the Exercises

Variant One: Chair Pose

Step 1 (Starting Position): Sit down on a chair, facing a wall if it helps you stay straight. Your back should be aligned, your hands and legs relaxed. Look straight ahead.

Step 2: Bring your hands on your knees, palms facing upward. Connect your thumb to your index finger.

Step 3: Close your eyes, inhale in, and exhale out. Be completely present at the moment.

Step 4: Continue breathing in and out ten times.

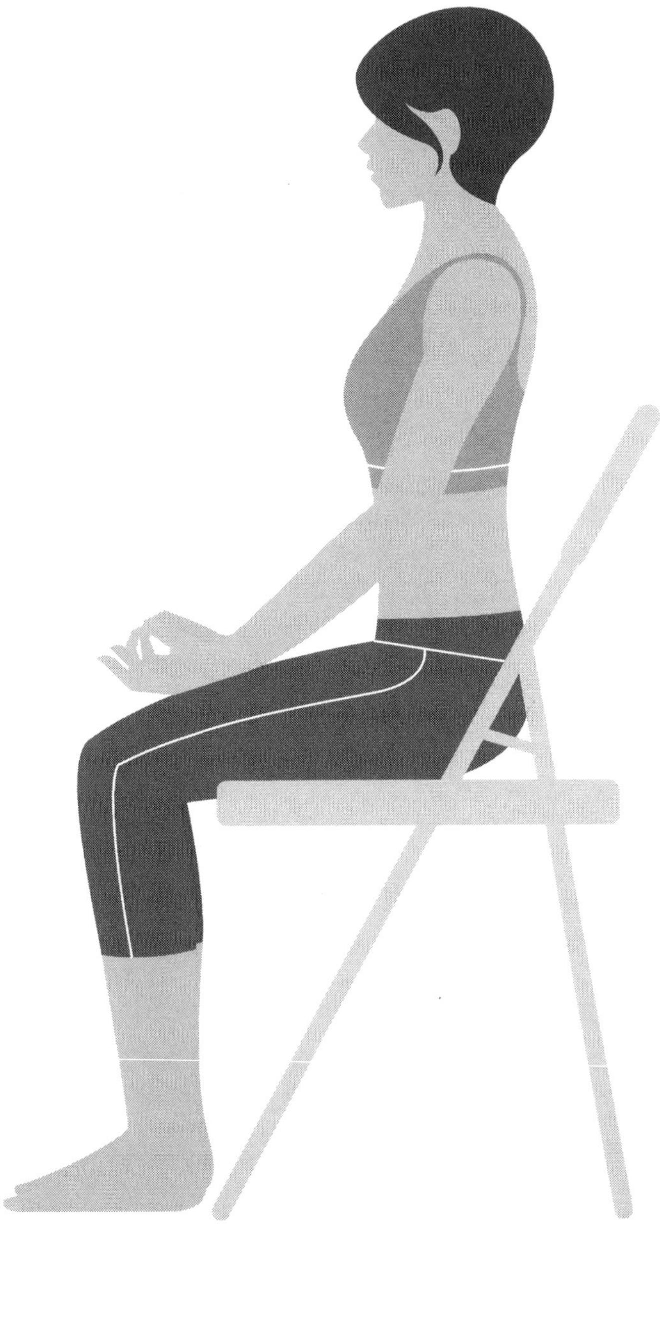

Variant Two: Sun Salutations

Step 1 (Starting Position): Be seated on a chair, palms on your knees, straight posture, eyes facing forward.

Step 2: Gently raise both your hands above your head in a circular motion, and touch your palms as if you are doing a pranam. Breathe in when you are raising your hands. Breathe out when your palms touch.

Step 3: Gently lower your hands in an anticlockwise motion, and return them to your knees.

Step 4: Repeat ten times.

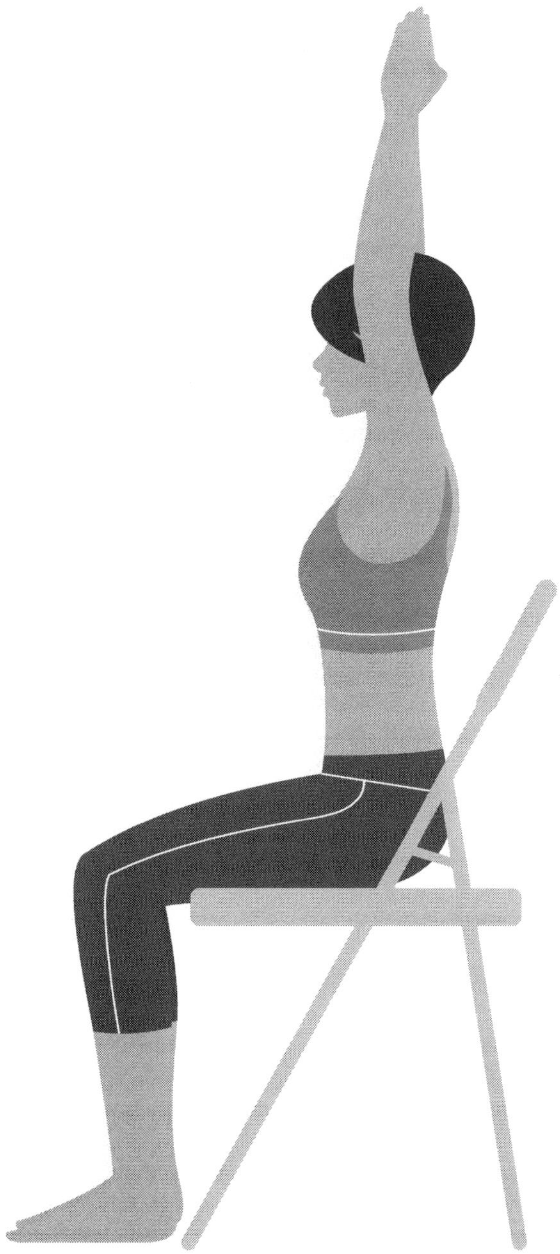

Variant Three: Forward Bend with Arm Extension

Step 1 (Starting Position): Sit straight on a chair, with your eyes facing forward and back aligned. Keep your hands neutral.

Step 2: Raise your hands in front of you in a vertical motion and extend them fully. Touch your palms together.

Step 3: Lower your head from your shoulders until your upper torso is in between your arms. Pause. Breathe in while you lower your head; breathe out once your torso is lowered.

Step 4: Gently return to the starting position. Neutralize your arms.

Step 5: Repeat this process ten times.

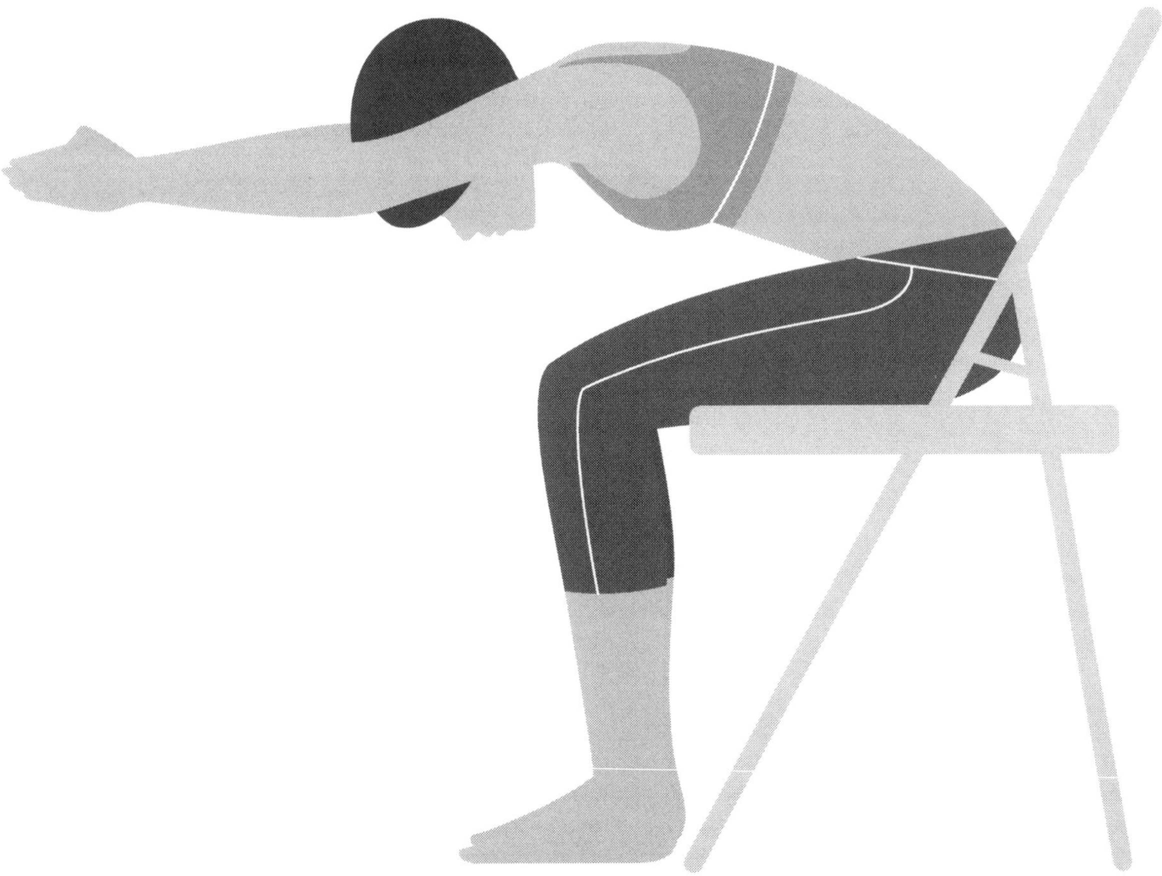

Variant Four: Forward Bend with Clasped Elbows

Step 1 (Starting Position): Sit straight with your arms by your sides, eyes looking ahead.

Step 2: Raise your hands vertically in front of you and clasp the left elbow with your right palm and the right elbow with your left palm.

Step 3: Lower your head from your shoulders. Stop when your upper torso is vertically positioned between your arms. Breathe in as you lower yourself and slowly breathe out once you reach the position.

Step 4: Return to the starting position.

Step 5: Repeat ten times.

Things to Remember:

- Always keep your back straight. Facing a wall may help you to be in a neutral position.
- Remember to keep your eyes in front of you. If you lower them, you might slouch, and if you keep them too high, you may arch your back. This will undo the benefits of the exercise. For maximum benefit, always keep your level.
- Breathing is a critical component of yoga, so always inhale and exhale at every point.
- Challenge yourself. If ten repetitions seem easy, increase them to 155–20. If it seems too much, do five repetitions and increase as you get stronger.

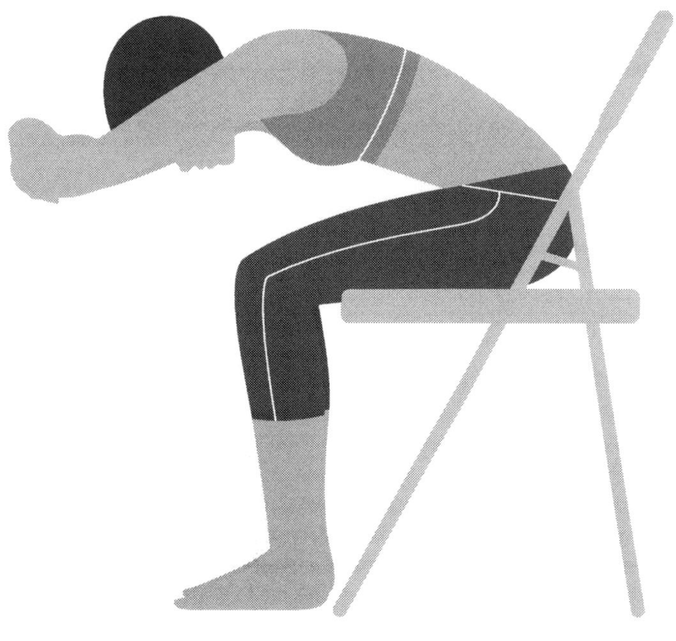

Yoga for Hip and Lower Back Pain

Yoga is a mind-body treatment that's often used for treating back pain and the tension that comes with it. The right poses will help you relax while still strengthening your body. Only a few minutes of yoga practice every day will help you become aware of your body. This will help you notice where you're tense and where your balance is failing you. You can use this knowledge to re-establish harmony and alignment in your life. If you have complaints about lower back pain, it's possible that your hips are to blame. These ten poses will help you strengthen all the correct muscles and address the root of your pain.

Start by making it a routine to get up and walk around for a few minutes to combat this issue. Then, as part of your everyday routine, integrate this yoga program. It will help you strengthen your hips, which will help you fight lower back pain. Let's talk about some simple yoga postures you can incorporate into your routine.

Seated Figure Four Exercise

Seated Figure Four is a simple Yoga posture that will help you ease the muscles of your back and hips. It also stretches the piriformis and glutes and relieves stress in the sacral muscles. The piriformis, which stretches from the base of the spine to the top of the femur and aids in hip rotation and stabilization, is the muscle situated deep in your glutes. The piriformis should be kept mobile to avoid inflammation or compression of the sciatic nerve.

Particulars:

Difficulty Level: Easy

Equipment Needed: None

Repetitions: 20 repetitions for 2 sets.

Performing the Exercise:

Step 1 (Starting Position): Sit on the floor with your knees bent and your feet flat on the floor.

Step 2: Cross your left ankle directly above your knee on top of your right thigh. Make a left-foot flex.

Step 3: Sit tall and inhale. Bring your hips closer to your right foot for a longer stretch.

Step 4: Hold your breath for ten seconds, release, and repeat.

Things to Remember:

- Keep your breathing even, and remember to inhale and exhale at every point.
- Make sure you are not feeling uncomfortable with any of the steps. This will undo the purpose of the exercise.
- If you can hold the stretch longer than ten seconds, go for it. But if ten seconds is too much, begin with five.

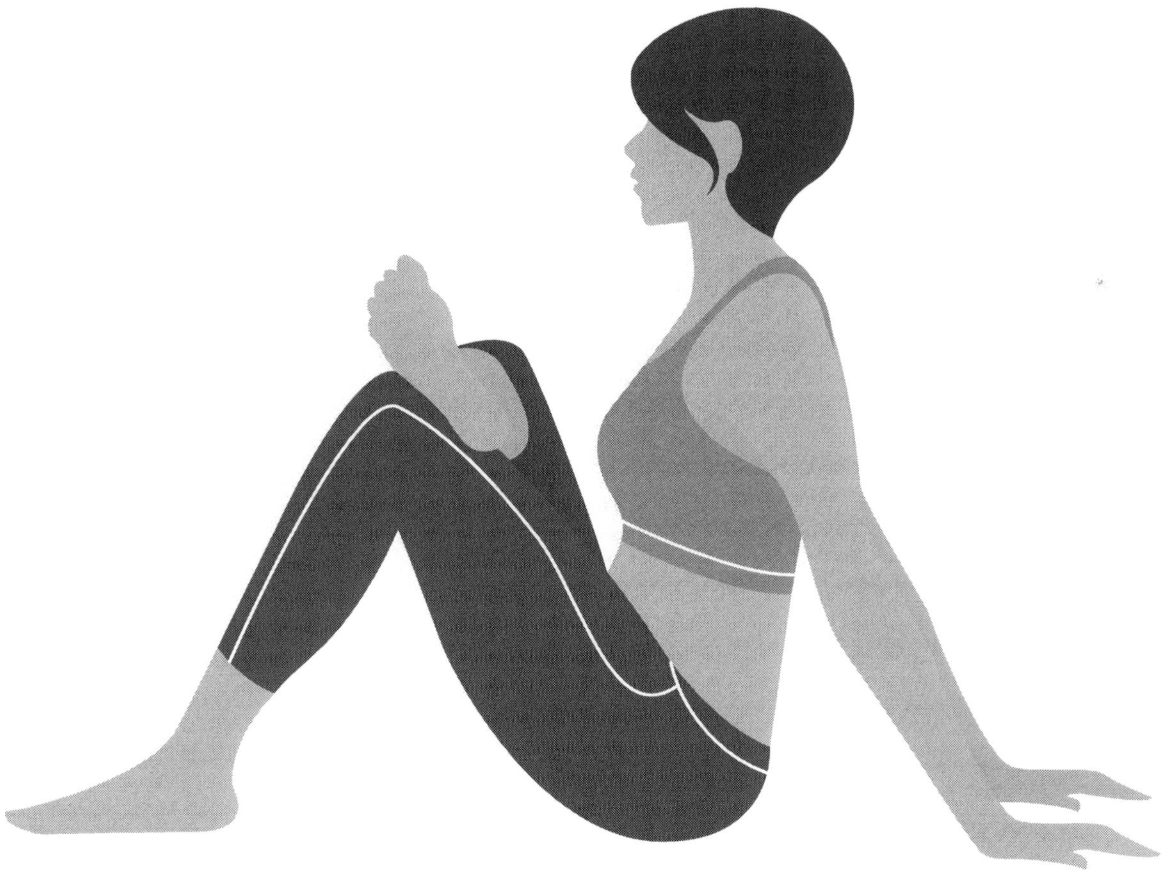

Crescent Lunge with Prayer Hands

This is a great yoga pose to enhance your overall flexibility. It increases balance and strength, stretches your lungs, back, abdomen, neck, shoulders, and groin. It also strengthens your calves, ankles, and thighs.

Particulars:

Difficulty Level: Advanced

Equipment Needed: None

Repetitions: 10 repetitions.

Performing the Exercise:

Step 1 (Starting Position): Exhale and take a step forward with your right foot between your hands. Align your right knee over your heel. Then, while keeping your right knee fixed in place, lower your left knee to the floor and slide your left back until you feel a relaxed stretch in your left front thigh.

Step 2: Inhale and straighten your torso. Raise your pubic bone toward your navel and draw your tailbone back toward the floor.

Step 3: Place your hands in front of your chest in a prayer position. Maintain a forward gaze.

Step 4: Take a deep inhalation, and press back to the starting point.

Step 5: Repeat.

Things to Remember:

- This yoga pose is advanced and requires a fair amount of balance, so go easy on yourself if it takes time.
- Keep your breathing even.
- Don't arch your back or push too hard. Only do as much as is comfortable.

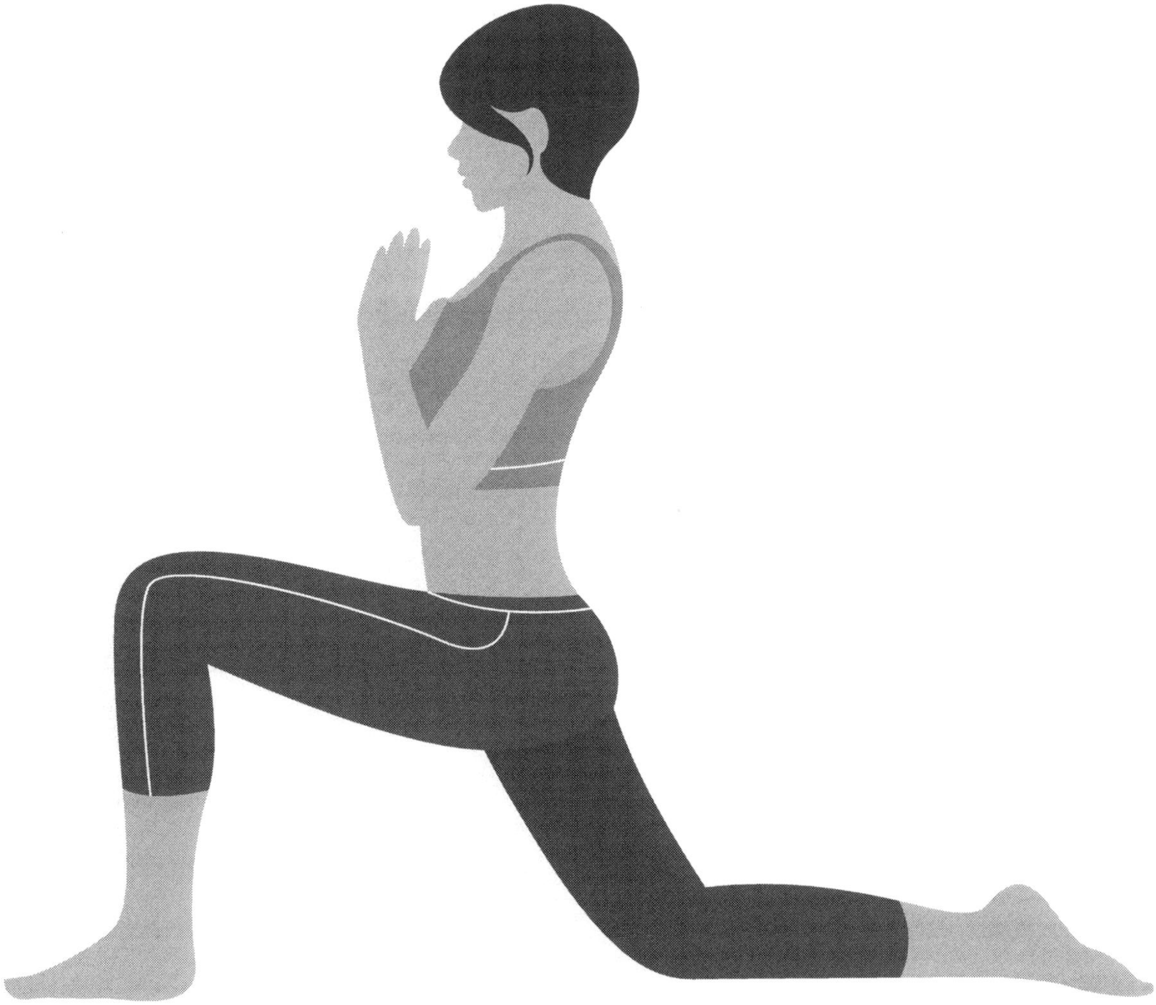

Yoga for Stiff and Tight Legs

Once you start yoga, you'll realize that many of the poses are difficult not because of the pose itself but because it requires you to hold an immense amount of balance in your legs. The effort can even make your legs shake. This allows your leg muscles to become activated and stronger. In 2014, a study looked at the effects of Hatha Yoga (a variant of yoga for your legs and whole body) compared with calisthenics in older adults. The study lasted for a year, after which the researchers noted that Hatha Yoga was far more effective in increasing balance and flexibility. With this, let's look at some yoga poses that will make your legs stronger and allow you to move around freely and without fear of falling (Farinatti et al., 2014).

Downward Facing Dog

This is one of the most practiced and basic yoga poses, particularly if you are just starting. It stretches your hamstrings, calves, lower back, and glutes. Its versatility is immense as it works on your shoulders and upper back!

Particulars:

Difficulty Level: Easy

Equipment Needed: None

Repetitions: 60-second repetitions done five times.

Performing the Exercise:

Step 1 (Starting Position): Start by getting down on your hands and knees. A yoga mat may be used for help.

Step 2: Ensure that your hands are directly under your shoulders and that your feet are directly beneath your hips. Keep your core engaged.

Step 3: Take a deep breath and raise yourself off your knees by pressing your weight into your palms, tucking your toes under. Hands should be shoulder-width apart, and heels should be hip-width apart.

Step 4: Lengthen your spine and tailbone. Keep your hands on the ground. On both sides of the body, your weight should be equally distributed.

Step 5: It's perfectly fine if there's any distance between your heels and the floor. Keep this pose for 1 minute, pressing both heels as hard as you can without straining.

Things to Remember:

- Examine the toes. From your elbows to your hips, your body should be in a straight line.
- Maintain a straight line with your arms and do not lock your elbows. Your legs should also be straight.
- Keep your breathing even.

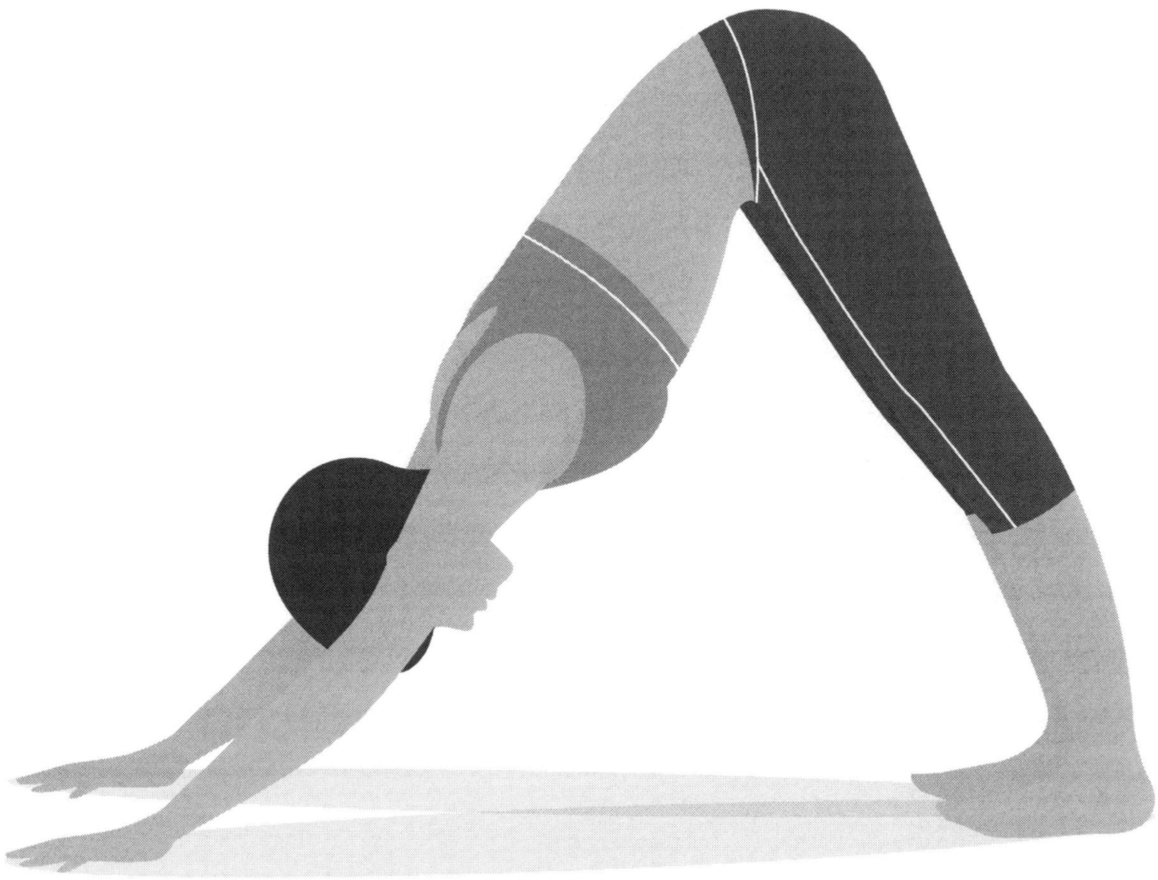

Lunge Pose

This is essentially a low lunge, which is beneficial for stretching your quads, hamstrings, and groin. It is a great way to release the tension in your hips.

Particulars:

Difficulty Level: Intermediate

Equipment Needed: None

Repetitions: 5 deep breaths on each leg. Repeat on each leg four times.

Performing the Exercise:

Step 1 (Starting Position): Go down on all fours in a high plank.

Step 2: Gently and slowly take your left leg ahead and rest it between your hands. Make sure that the right leg is straight backward.

Step 3: Press through your right foot as you press your palms into the floor.

Step 4: Take your shoulders back and breathe through your chest, arching forward just a little.

Step 5: Take five deep breaths and step back with your left leg. Repeat on the other side.

Things to Remember:

- This one can be tricky in terms of balance, so don't feel bad if you fumble. Just go slow.
- Keep your breathing even.
- Make sure that your core is engaged and that your legs are working throughout the exercise.

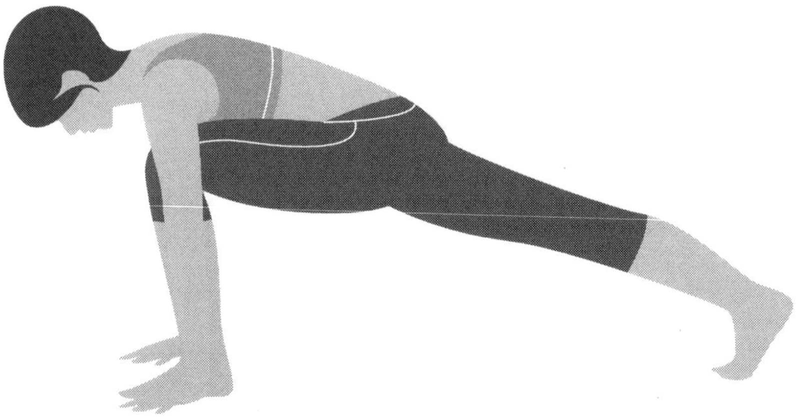

Half-Splits

Half Splits Pose is a gentle way to open up the legs for people of all ages. The calves, hamstrings, and groin are stretched in Half Splits Pose. They also aid in the correction of posture and breathing and the relief of joint pain.

Particulars:

Difficulty Level: Intermediate

Equipment Needed: None

Repetitions: Inhale and exhale for 10 seconds on each leg. Repeat on each leg five times.

Performing the Exercise:

Step 1 (Starting Position): Start in Downward-Facing Dog, with your palms firmly planted on the floor and your hips lifted high and back. Take a few deep breaths while bending your knees and raising your heels to loosen up the back of your thighs.

Step 2: Move your right foot forward between your hands on an exhale. Lower your left knee to the ground and release the top of your left foot.

Step 3: Straighten your right leg as much as you can by flexing your right foot, coming up onto the heel, and extending your toes back toward you.

Step 4: Maintain a squared-off posture with your hips stacked over your left leg. Inhale to lengthen your back, then exhale and fold your right leg.

Step 5: Draw your right heel back and forward when reaching your chest forward and your shoulder blades down and away from your face.

Step 6: Stay in the pose for ten seconds. Tuck the left toes under, plant the hands, and return to Downward-Facing Dog to come out of the pose. When you're ready, switch sides and repeat.

Things to Remember:

- If having your hands on the ground feels too difficult, try walking your hands closer to your body or elevating your hands on blocks to reduce the stretch's strength.
- If your back knee is bothering you, consider using a mat and tucking a blan ket or towel under it for extra support.

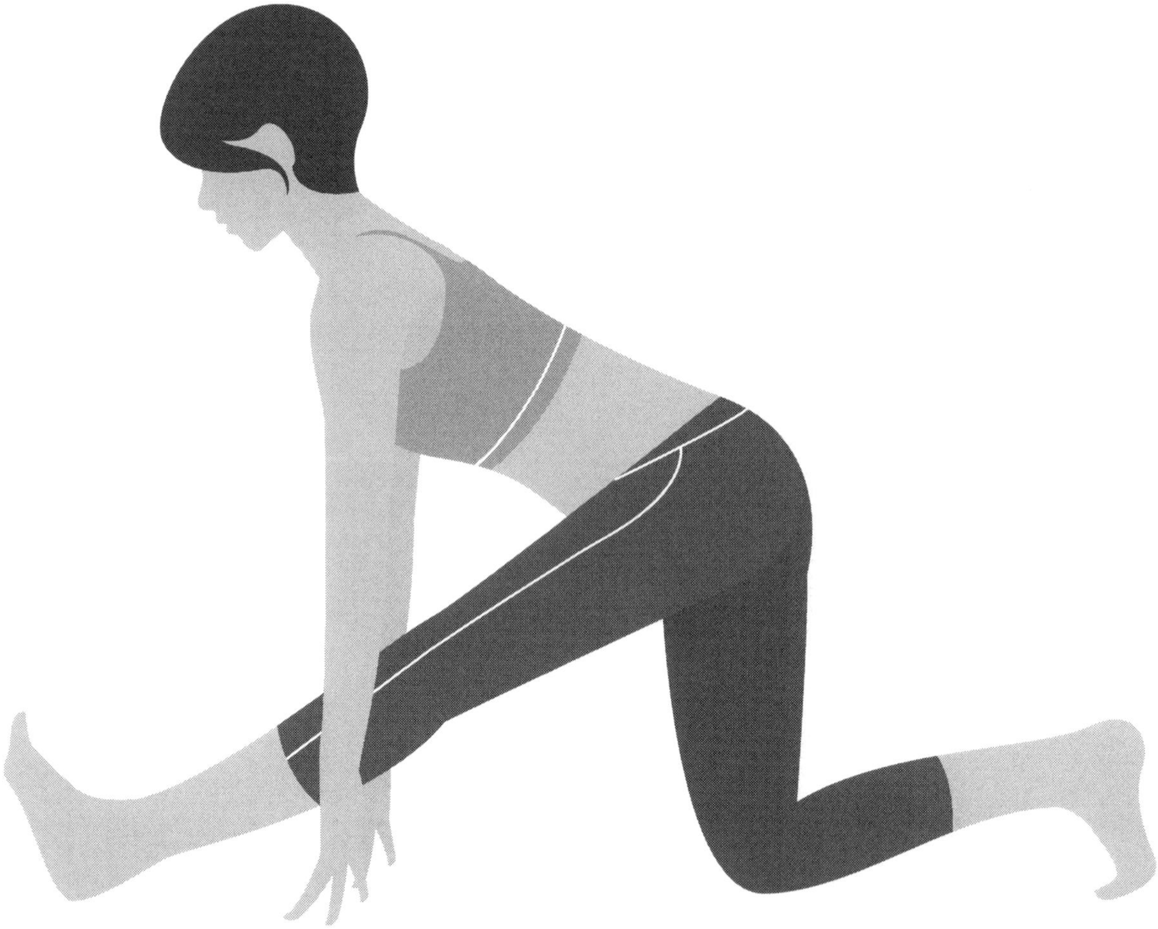

Halfway Lift

Stretch your hamstrings, your upper back, and lengthen your entire spine with this soothing pose. It will require practice and balance, so work your way into it slowly.

Particulars:

Difficulty Level: Advanced

Equipment Needed: None

Repetitions: 10-second-deep breaths at the end pose. Repeat exercise ten times.

Performing the Exercise:

Step 1 (Starting Position): When you stand, bend over while holding your spine erect. Your feet should be shoulder-width apart or hip-width apart.

Step 2: Place your fingertips next to your feet on the ground. Put your palms to your shins with your fingers pointing straight down.

Step 3: Straighten your arms and raise your shoulders away from your thighs as you inhale. Lengthen your spine and slightly contract your upper back muscles.

Step 4: Look ahead slightly without craning your neck.

Step 5: Maintain a solid center and stop rounding the spine. If bending your knees lets you find more length, do so.

Step 6: Release back into the standing forward bend as you exhale.

Things to Remember:

- This is difficult only in terms of how much balance it needs. It requires you to bend, so be gentle with yourself.
- If you have trouble bending, do not attempt this pose.

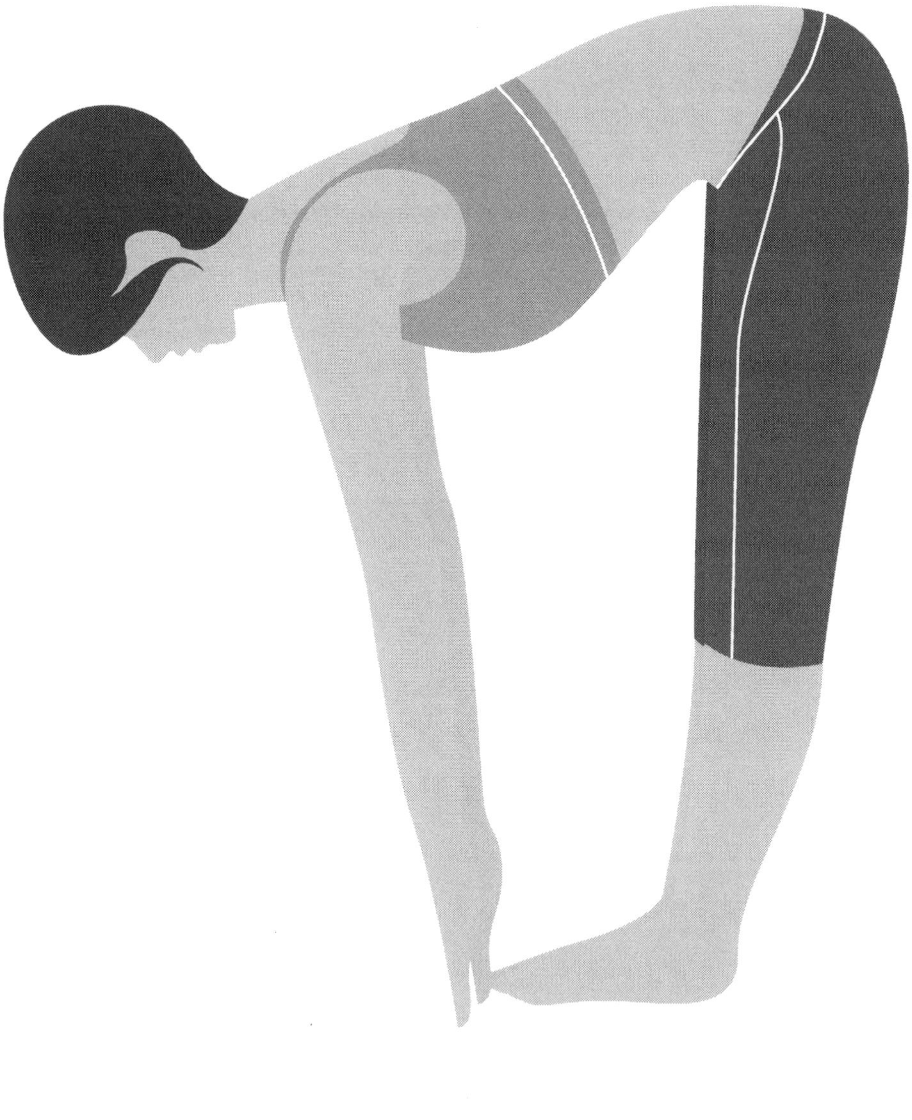

Yoga for Lower Back Tension

Yoga is one of the most common ways to alleviate low back pain and tension. The practice helps strengthen muscles that support the back and neck, including the spinal muscles, which help you bend your spine, the multifidus muscles, which stabilize your vertebrae, and the transversus abdominis muscle, which helps stabilize your spine. Many of the postures in yoga are designed to strengthen the back and abdominal muscles gently. The muscular network of the spine includes back and abdominal muscles, which help the body maintain proper upright posture and movement. Back pain and tension can be significantly minimized or eliminated when these muscles are well-conditioned.

Cow Pose

This simple, straightforward exercise is gentle on your body. It stretches and mobilizes your spine and also stretches the shoulders, torso, and neck. It works on the erector spinae, triceps, gluteus maximus, rectus abdominis, and serratus anterior muscles.

Particulars:

Difficulty Level: Easy

Equipment Needed: None

Repetitions: Breath for 40 seconds at each repetition. Repeat ten times.

Performing the Exercise:

Step 1 (Starting Position)

Begin in a "tabletop" position on your hands and knees.

Ensure that your knees are directly behind your hips and that your wrists, elbows, and shoulders are in line with the floor.

With your eyes on the floor, position your head neutrally.

Step 2: Inhale. Raise your chest toward the ceiling as you inhale, allowing your belly to sag to the floor. Lift your brows and look straight ahead.

Step 3: Exhale and return to your hands and knees in a neutral "tabletop" spot.

Step 4: Repeat.

Things to Remember:

- Never bounce on this movement because you may end up injuring your neck.
- Be in control of the movement and keep your eyes focused ahead of you.

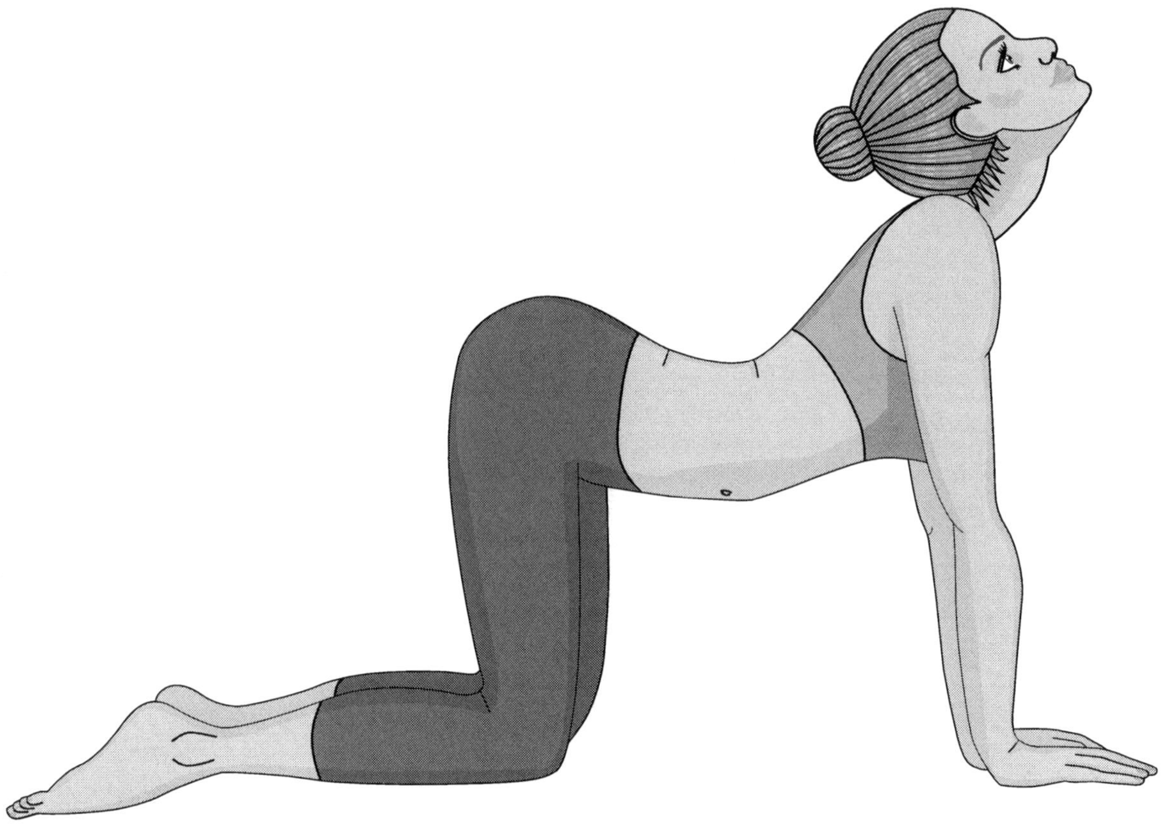

The Cat Pose

A variant of the Cow pose, this posture massages the spine and abdominal organs gently. It is a great way to ease your back, particularly if you have chronic back issues.

Particulars:

Difficulty Level: Easy

Equipment Needed: None

Repetitions: Breath for 40 seconds at each repetition. Repeat ten times.

Performing the Exercise:

Step 1 (Starting Position):

Begin in a "tabletop" position on your hands and knees.

Ensure that your knees are directly behind your hips and that your wrists, elbows, and shoulders are in line with the floor.

Keep your head in a neutral position with your eyes on the ground.

Step 2: Round your spine toward the ceiling as you exhale, keeping your shoulders and knees in place. Allow your head to fall to the floor, but keep your chin from collapsing into your stomach. Breathe.

Step 3: Return to a neutral "tabletop" position on your hands and knees by inhaling.

Step 4: Repeat.

Things to Remember:

- As with the cow pose, keep your eyes fixed and go through the movement as gently as possible.
- Don't forget to breathe.

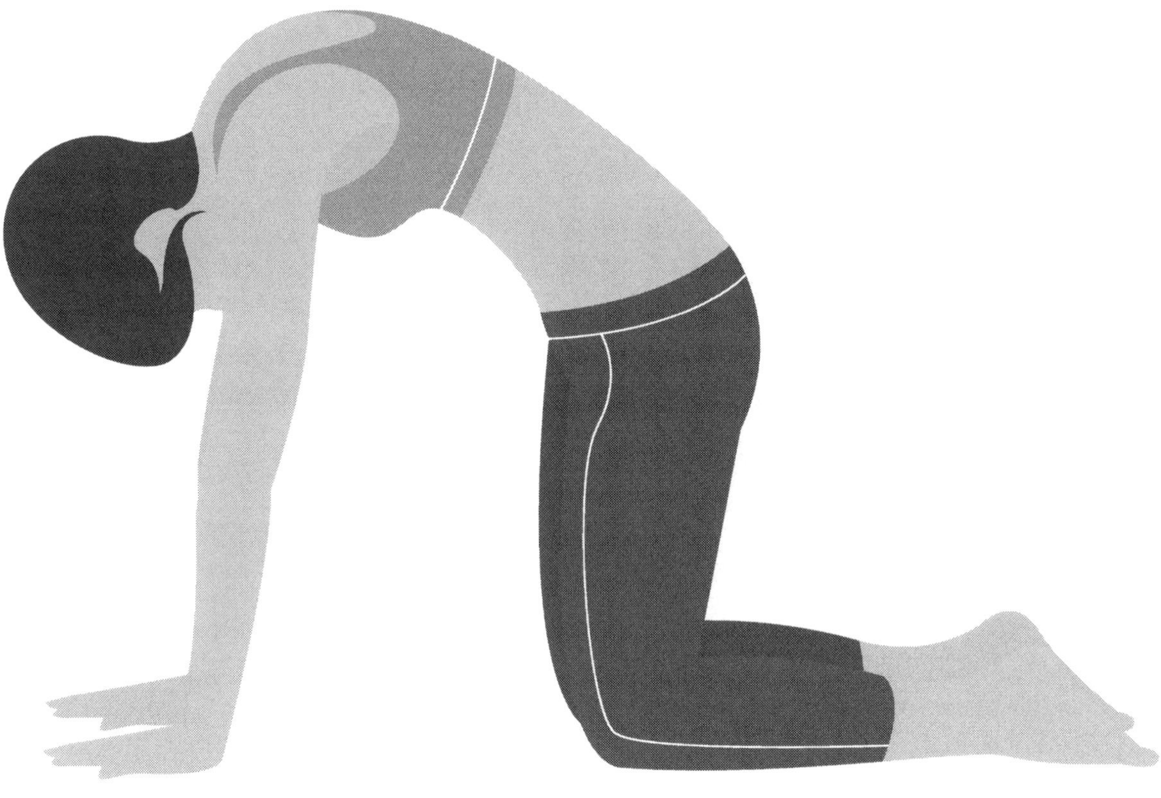

Side Body Stretch

The Side Stretch Pose increases energy levels in the body. It relaxes the lower back, mid-back, biceps and triceps, core (abs), hip flexors, Hips, neck, pelvis, Erector spinae, and quadriceps.

Particulars:

Difficulty Level: Intermediate

Equipment Needed: None

Repetitions: Hold each rep for 40 seconds. Repeat 20 times.

Performing the Exercise:

Step 1 (Starting Position): Sit with your legs crossed. Keep your left hand on the floor, keeping the elbow bent.

Step 2: Extend your right arm upwards and over your head.

Step 3: Move your arms from the right to the left until you feel a stretch to your right.

Step 4: Hold here for 40 seconds, return to starting position, and repeat.

Things to Remember:

- Don't overextend your right hand. Do it until you feel a good stretch.
- Don't arch your back; your spine should be straight and neutral. Learn from your hips.
- Keep your breathing even.

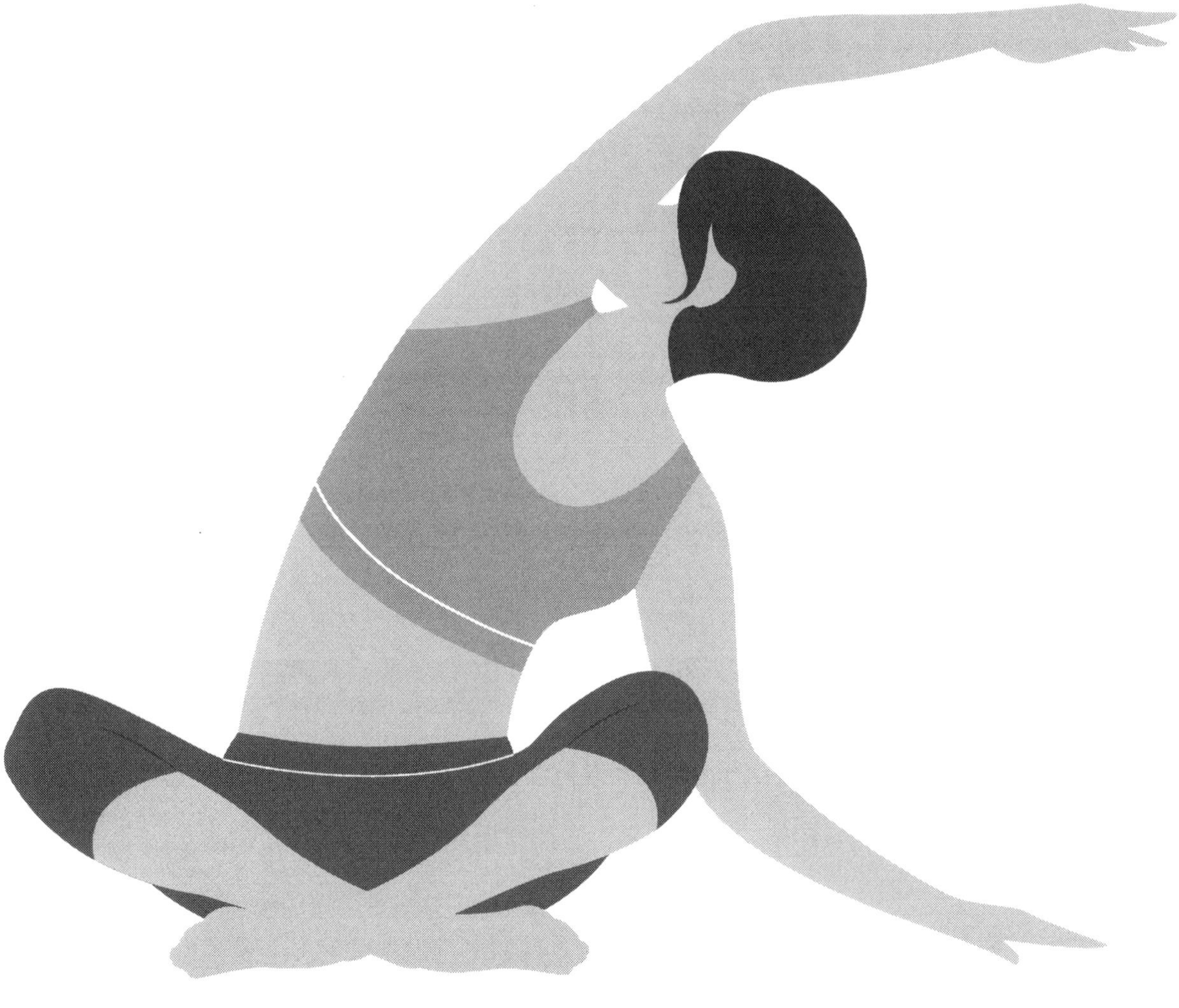

Seated Twist Pose

This variation of the seated stretch allows you to get a deeper stretch into your muscles while increasing your balance and endurance.

Particulars:

Difficulty Level: Advanced

Equipment Needed: None

Repetitions: Hold each rep for 40 seconds. Repeat 20 times.

Performing the Exercise:

Step 1 (Starting Position): Sit with your legs crossed. Keep your left hand on the floor, keeping the elbow bent.

Step 2: Extend your right arm behind and keep extending it until it reaches your left hip. You will find yourself twisting. Twist from your core.

Step 3: Bring your left hand and rest the palm on your right knee.

Step 4: Move yourself from the right to the left until you feel a stretch.

Step 5: Hold here for 40 seconds, return to starting position, and repeat.

Things to Remember:

- Don't overextend your arm. Just do as much as is comfortable.
- Remember that the arm you are reaching back has to turn towards the hip of the other side.
- This will take time to master since the exercise is a deep one. Be patient.

Chapter 4: **Balance Exercises**

Discovering balance in all aspects of your life is the way forward. This remembers creating balance for your body.

Further developing equilibrium builds coordination and strength, permitting you to move openly and consistently. Improving steadiness, versatility, and adaptability makes it simpler to play out your day-by-day errands. It likewise works on your athletic presentation. Zeroing in on your equilibrium may likewise assist you with centering and clear your brain.

How Balance Exercises Work

Adjusting practices work your center muscles, lower back, and legs. Lower-body strength-preparing activities can likewise assist with working in your equilibrium.

While adjusting activities can be trying on occasion, predictable exertion will make these activities simpler. The number of redundancies increments step by step as the activities become simpler. You might request that somebody direct or help you, particularly when you're initially beginning.

You can change the activities to increment or decline the trouble or adapt to your requirements. Start on your non-dominant side with the goal that the subsequent side is simpler. You can do your non-dominant side twice, assuming you need to adjust your body between the two sides. When you become familiar with the activities, take a stab at doing them with one of the two eyes shut.

Balance Exercises for Seniors

These activities keep your body dynamic, further develop equilibrium and coordination, and forestall falls and wounds.

Rock the Boat

Remain with your feet hip-width separated.

Press your weight into the two feet immovably and equitably.

Put your weight onto your left foot and lift your right foot.

Hold for as long as 30 seconds.

Gradually lower your left foot to the floor and do the same on the other side.

Do each side five to multiple times.

Joined Triplanar Toe Taps

Put an obstruction band around your lower thighs, simply over your knees.

Come into a solitary leg, quarter-squat on your right leg.

Draw in your center and hips muscles.

Utilizing the opposition of the band, tap your left leg forward, aside, and straight behind you.

Do 10 to 20 reiterations.

Then, at that point, do the contrary side.

Single-Leg Cross-Body Punches

Hold two free weights at chest tallness.

Lean your weight onto your left foot, coming into a quarter-squat.

Keeping your left leg solid and stable, punch the loads across your body, each in turn.

Then, at that point, do the contrary side.

Do one to three arrangements of 10 to 20 redundancies.

Paloff Press with Rotation

Stand confronting a link machine.

Utilizing two hands, hold the link handles at the stature of your chest.

Stroll to the right side and broaden your arms from your body.

Connect with your center as you get some distance from the machine, keeping up with arrangement through the middle line of your body.

Keep your arms stretched out and get back to the beginning position.

Then, at that point, do the contrary side.

Do up 1 to 3 arrangements of 10 to 20 reiterations.

Balance Exercises for Parkinson's Disease

Rehearsing your balance is indispensable in the event that you have Parkinson's illness since it assists with expanding strength and perseverance. You can likewise evaluate a portion of these yoga stances to work on your portability, and, by and large, personal satisfaction.

Chair Leg Raises

To expand the trouble, this activity should be possible with a lower leg weight.

Sit in a seat with a straight spine and the two feet straightforwardly under your knees.

Gradually, fix your left leg, holding it up for a couple of moments.

Lower it back down and rehash with your right leg.

Do up to 1 to 3 arrangements of 10 to 20 reiterations.

Side-Stepping

From a standing position, step sideways to the right half of the room.

Lift your knees as high as possible while moving like you're venturing over something.

Then, at that point, get back to one side of the room.

Why Balance Is Significant

Further developed balance makes day-by-day exercises, like strolling on steps, conveying weighty things, and out of nowhere adjusting bearings simpler. A strong, stable base will permit you to move with more coordination, straightforwardness, and smoothness. You'll likewise acquire more grounded and more upgraded development during athletic exercises.

Growing great equilibrium assists with working on your general wellbeing and wellness levels. These enhancements help to forestall the danger of injury and fall, particularly in more established grown-ups and individuals with Parkinson's illness. This permits you to keep up with your freedom longer.

Stay mindful of your stance and strength for the duration of the day. Notice in case you're yielding your weight uniformly on the two feet and work to root your weight into your feet.

You can likewise focus on whether you will, in general, yield your body weight forward or in reverse in space. Attempt to bring your body into a legitimate arrangement and feel a solid association with the floor. Notice where and how you lose your equilibrium and make the suitable redress in your body.

Chapter 5: **Basics of Nutritional Science That You Need to Know**

Calories

These are often demonized, but calories are just a measure of the energy that you get from eating and digesting a portion of food. This doesn't mean it's healthy or unhealthy—what's unhealthy is getting the wrong quantity of calories for your goal in a day or a week.

Calories only tell us what happens with weight, not what that weight is or what it does. Eating more calories than you use in a day means you're going to gain weight (as either muscle or fat) while eating less than you use in a day means you're going to lose weight (again, either as muscle or fat).

The amount you use in a day is an estimate called the Total Daily Energy Expenditure (TDEE), and we use this as our starting point for how much we need to eat in a day. You can log your food with mobile apps like MyFitnessPal to keep track of what you eat throughout the day.

This kind of tracking is awesome because, if nothing else, you'll come to understand what is in certain foods. This can be a huge part of the dietary process, showing you where you're over-eating, often without even knowing it!

People "on a diet" tend to restrict calories, as this is how you achieve fat loss, while muscle-gain diets are usually in a calorie surplus. Setting your own goals is key here to make sure you're getting the right quantity of calories.

You usually want to be around 300 to 500 calories above or below your TDEE. More than 500 under tends to be too restrictive and can cause more muscle loss, while more than 500 calories over the TDEE will likely cause more fat gain than intended.

These are also great lines for keeping progress sustainable and being able to commit to the process for an extended period of time. They also match up with the progress speed I mentioned above: 500 calories under your TDEE every day will produce around 1lb of fat loss per week or around 0.5lb of muscle gain.

Macros

Macronutrients are the major building blocks of food and are the most plentiful nutrients within it, hence the name. There are three macronutrients that each have an important role in the diet:

Proteins are one of the building blocks of cells and are primarily used in the body to repair or build crucial tissues, with muscle being one of those. Bones, tendons, muscles, and organs are all heavily dependent on proteins—more of them in the diet means better metabolism, better muscle growth, and prioritizing fat-burning when we eat under our TDEE.

Carbohydrates are the main short- and mid-term energy source for the body. They include sugars and starches, as well as the non-digestible fiber, which is key for metabolic and digestive health. Carbs are going to make up a decent portion of the diet and what matters is the quality of source you choose. Ideally, this means more starches and fiber, especially from pulses and whole grains.

Fats are important for cell membranes, keeping the brain healthy (especially as you age), and helping with hormonal health. They're more calorie-dense than either protein or carbs, so you want to get less of them. They're also long-term energy sources for when you run out of carbohydrates in the body.

Micros

Micronutrients are vitamins and minerals—they're not any less important. They just don't tend to have calorie values. Your body doesn't use them for energy or as the building blocks of tissues, but they do play secondary and supporting roles in these processes, and you're going to run into major health risks if you're deficient in vitamins and minerals.

It's easy to look at it in an oversimplified way: micronutrients are all about health. They relate to things like performance results, but they're mostly important for keeping your organs healthy and functioning as intended.

There are 25 essential vitamins and minerals that you need to focus on, but they're all provided through a combination of lean proteins, choosing the right carb sources (like pulses and whole grains), and then a good quantity and variety of fruits and veg.

There are 12 essential vitamins:

- A
- B1
- B2
- B3
- B6
- B7
- B9
- B12
- C
- D
- E
- K

And 13 essential minerals:

- Iron
- Calcium
- Sodium
- Potassium
- Magnesium
- Zinc
- Iron
- Copper
- Manganese
- Phosphorus
- Chromium
- Iodine

These are a lot to remember, but just note that they're the ones to focus on. What we want to do is avoid deficiency, which is primarily done by eating the kind of diet outlined above, but also through the variety and range of plant foods in the diet.

Focus should go specifically to getting lots of B vitamins, vitamin D, and minerals like magnesium, potassium, and iron. It's definitely worth getting your vitamin and mineral levels checked with your doctor whenever possible so you can look at what specifically is missing from your diet.

Food Quality

As we get through the basics, you can start looking at your sources of carbs and vitamins and minerals. Some sources are better than others for their concentration of pseudo-vitamins, but more specifically, we're looking to focus on whole foods.

These are the kinds of "real foods" we want in the diet because they tend to contain fiber, better ratios of proteins to fats, and they're usually more nutrient-dense. What you want to avoid is demonizing non-whole foods, though.

Some foods are specifically designed to get the best of a whole food or are refined in ways that simply make them better to eat without compromising the nutritional or health qualities of the food. The idea is to get whole foods into the diet wherever possible and avoid depending on non-whole foods.

This is a good thing to work on in the long run, but it should not be your focus until you've already gotten your calories and macronutrients in place. Many people fail their diets by rushing straight to this step and ignoring the more important stuff above!

Food Timing

You can get a little more benefit out of your food if you eat it at specific times. This is a step beyond food selection, and it's where you really start getting into the fine details. It's not something you need to worry about too much, but here's a quick overview.

Carbs are better consumed closer to exercise and consumed less further away from exercise and activity. Specifically, Sugars are best consumed very near exercise or even during to keep your energy levels up and maintain glucose levels during exercise. This has been related to improved performance and is the best time to get in that sugary snack you're in love with.

Proteins are best dosed regularly through the day, if possible, but specifically after exercise and activity. Post-workout meals should focus on proteins and carbohydrates, as these are the resources that exercise depletes, and eating them supports the systems that repair and develop muscles and tendons.

Fats should be consumed even further out of exercise than carbohydrates since they're a slower source of energy and can often sit heavily. We want to reduce but not eliminate fat intake around the time of exercise to keep the digestive system happy, saving fats for breakfasts and evening meals after our workouts.

Supplements

You don't need supplements, but they can provide a great helping hand for a diet—whatever level you're at. Even if you're mastering the diet and putting 100% effort in, you can benefit from strategic supplement use.

We see this in elite athletes: people whose diets are perfect, but they're still using multivitamins, protein supplements, creatine, and cod liver oil, as well as an effervescent. These are the kinds of supplements you should look at.

Supplements allow you to top up your diet with compounds important for performance and health in a convenient way. They're ways of improving your intake without having to eat a ridiculous number of fish, beef, or eggs, for example.

This is when concentrated sources are great—but, again, you shouldn't use them to replace a shortcoming in your diet. The idea is that they are supplementary: they're added on top of a good and developing diet, but they're not a replacement for good dietary habits.

A diet isn't just a collection of scientific principles about metabolism and nutrients. It's a habit change that has a person in the middle of it—and these factors need to be considered because they're going to be about your experience on a diet.

After all, science doesn't do the work for you: simply knowing what you need to do doesn't make it happen. That comes from the hard work of being self-aware with your diet and working on the bits that you're bad at, improving your habits day by day, and making good choices when that cake is calling to you.

Remember that dieting is a fallible process, and you're going to make mistakes—you're going to stumble, and you're going to have bad days. The ideal response is to just forget about it. You want to avoid anything like guilt or a spiral of "I've failed, may as well give up" that you see so often.

Chapter 6: **Seated Exercises**

Active Sitting

Active sitting helps us load our muscles and bones to fight the effects of gravity. Instead of outsourcing the role of our muscles by slumping in our seats, we should sit tall.

To start: Begin by sitting in a kitchen or dining room chair that has a firm seat.

Shifting forward: Slide your bottom forward, so you're not leaning back in the chair. Place both feet flat on the floor in front of you. If your legs are shorter and you can't touch the floor, you can place a large book or block on the floor to support your feet. Don't roll onto your tailbone. Imagine you have a tail, and you want the tail behind you so you can wag it. Often, people roll backward, so they're resting on their tailbone instead of their sit bones—these are the bony part of your bum, the lower edge of your pelvis.

Shoulder position: Drop your shoulders away from your ears. It should feel like you're letting them slide down your back.

Head position: Pull your head and neck back so your ears are sitting over your shoulders, not pushed forward. Your head is now positioned over your center of gravity, which is allowing you to strengthen your bones by loading them. Feel your muscles and bones at work.

Aim for five minutes of active sitting every hour.

Visualize: A string is tied to the top of your head, pulling you up towards the ceiling.

Do you need to make it easier? Start with two minutes of active sitting.

Are you ready to make it harder? Try for 10 minutes of active sitting every hour.

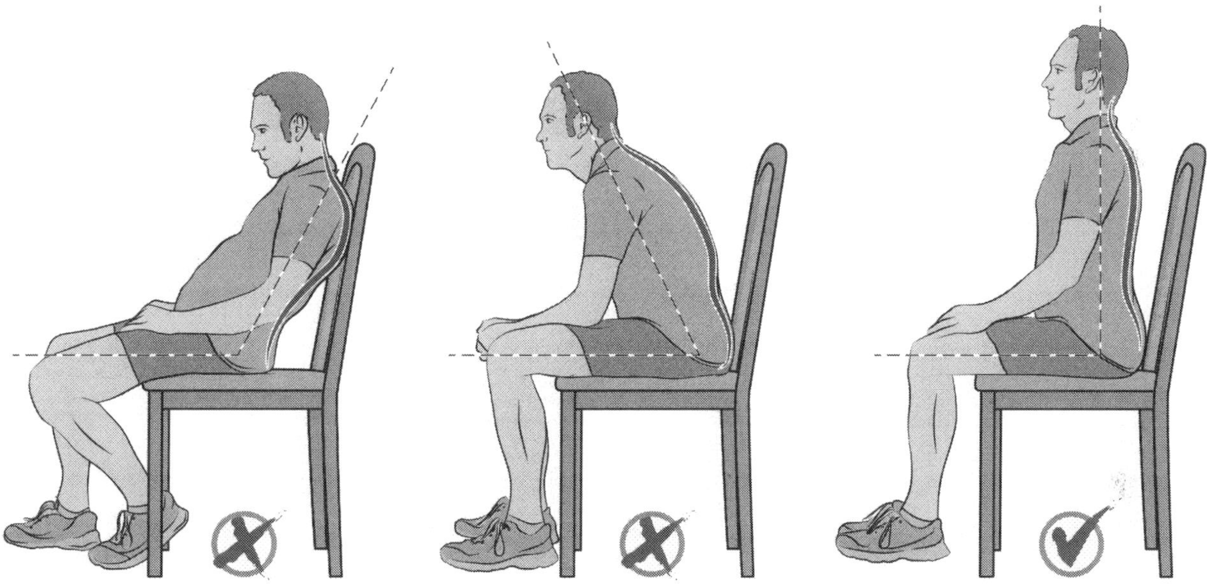

Seated Joint Mobility

CARs—Controlled Articular Rotations—involve making s-l-o-w, controlled circles that increase mobility in your joints. Drawing these circles helps you feel less stiff and move more fluidly. Remember, motion is lotion! Some of these joint mobility exercises can be completed standing, seated, or lying down and are thus repeated in the standing and lying down exercise. The key is to make slow and controlled movements. Many times, I see people drawing fast and sloppy circles. Fight the urge to get through the exercises as quickly as possible. Try to make the circular movements last for at least the number of seconds listed in the instructions.

Neck

To start: Sit comfortably in a chair. A dining room chair with no arms is best for optimal movement.

Clockwise: Looking straight ahead, rotate your head in a clockwise direction for five seconds.

Counterclockwise: Switch directions and repeat as you count another five seconds.

Visualize: The movement should look as if you're drawing a circle with the tip of your nose.

Do you need to make it easier? Count fewer seconds to complete the joint rotations, or repeat the sequence fewer times. Take breaks and rest.

Are you ready to make it harder? Please don't try to make it harder. CARs are a feel-good movement designed to keep your joints mobile. We don't want to force them to work harder, just better!

Shoulders

To start: Sit comfortably in a chair. A dining room chair with no arms is best for optimal movement.

Joint position: Relax your shoulders and keep your arms dropped at your side.

Forward: Slowly roll your shoulders forward, up, back, and down as you count to five.

Backward: Repeat in the opposite direction: pull them down, back, up, and forward as you count another five seconds.

Repeat: Repeat this sequence five to ten times.

Visualize: The movement should look as if your shoulders are a carpet that you are unrolling.

Do you need to make it easier? Count fewer seconds to complete the joint rotations, or repeat the sequence fewer times. Take breaks and rest.

Are you ready to make it harder? Please don't try to make it harder. CARs are a feel-good movement designed to keep your joints mobile. We don't want to force them to work harder, just better!

Elbows

To start: Sit comfortably in a chair. A dining room chair with no arms is best for optimal movement.

Joint position: Lift your arms out to the side at a slight angle. Bend your elbows so that your hands are pointing towards the floor.

Clockwise: Slowly make circles by rotating your lower arm—below the elbow—clockwise for five seconds.

Counterclockwise: Repeat in the other direction for another five seconds.

Repeat: Repeat this sequence five to ten times. Lower your arms to your sides when you are finished.

Visualize: Your arms look like a scarecrow, and the rest of your body is a tin man, so the only joint able to move in this position is your elbow. Your fingers are slowly drawing circles on the ground.

Do you need to make it easier? Count fewer seconds to complete the joint rotations, or repeat the sequence fewer times. Take breaks and rest.

Are you ready to make it harder? Please don't try to make it harder. CARs are a feel-good movement designed to keep your joints mobile. We don't want to force them to work harder, just better!

Wrists

To start: Sit comfortably in a chair. A dining room chair with no arms is best for optimal movement.

Joint position: Lift your hands in front of you at chest height.

Clockwise: Slowly rotate both of your wrists in a clockwise direction while you count to ten.

Counterclockwise: Slowly rotate your wrists in the opposite direction while you count to ten again.

Repeat: Repeat this sequence five to ten times. Lower your hands to your sides when you are finished.

Visualize: Two pots of jam are being held in front of you, and your hands are slowly stirring the thick spread.

Do you need to make it easier? Count fewer seconds to complete the joint rotations, or repeat the sequence fewer times. Take breaks and rest. Complete the movement as a lying down exercise.

Are you ready to make it harder? Please don't try to make it harder. CARs are a feel-good movement designed to keep your joints mobile. We don't want to force them to work harder, just better!

Fingers

To start: Sit comfortably in a chair. A dining room chair with no arms is best for optimal movement.

Joint position: Lift your hands in front of you and spread out your fingers. You will work both hands at the same time.

Clockwise: Starting with your pinky fingers, slowly draw circles with each pinky finger in a clockwise direction for five seconds.

Counterclockwise: Repeat in the opposite direction for five more seconds.

Repeat: Repeat circles in both directions with each finger. So, after you have finished with your pinky fingers, move on to your ring fingers, then your middle fingers, and your index fingers. When it's time to work your thumbs, slow down the circles even more. They have a bigger range of motion, so try to make circles with them for seven to eight seconds in each direction.

Visualize: Two pots of jam are being held in front of you, and your fingers are slowly stirring the thick spread.

Do you need to make it easier? Count fewer seconds to complete the joint rotations, or repeat the sequence fewer times. Take breaks and rest. Complete the movement as a lying down exercise.

Are you ready to make it harder? Please don't try to make it harder. CARs are a feel-good movement designed to keep your joints mobile. We don't want to force them to work harder, just better!

Waist

To start: Sit on the front edge of a chair with your feet planted on the ground. This will give you clearance to circle towards the back without hitting the back of your chair.

Clockwise: Slowly rotate your upper body in a clockwise circle as you count to five.

Counterclockwise: Repeat in a counterclockwise circle for five more seconds.

Repeat: Repeat this sequence five to ten times.

Visualize: You are a puppet, and the strings attached to your waist are being moved too slowly to lean you forwards and then back, in a circular pattern.

Do you need to make it easier? Count fewer seconds to complete the joint rotations, or repeat the sequence fewer times. Take breaks and rest.

Are you ready to make it harder? Please don't try to make it harder. CARs are a feel-good movement designed to keep your joints mobile. We don't want to force them to work harder, just better!

Ankles

To start: Sit comfortably in a chair.

Joint position: Lift your right foot off the ground and bend your knee.

Clockwise: Count to ten as you draw circles with your foot by rotating your ankle in a clockwise direction.

Counterclockwise: Count to ten as you draw circles in the opposite direction.

Repeat: Repeat this sequence five to ten times, then lower your right foot to the ground.

Other ankle: Lift your left foot off the ground and repeat the entire sequence in both directions, then lower your left foot to the ground.

You can even try wiggling your toes a little. These aren't rotations, just an additional feel-good movement.

Visualize: Your foot is a pencil, and you are using it to slowly draw circles on the ground.

Do you need to make it easier? Count fewer seconds to complete the joint rotations, or repeat the sequence fewer times. Take breaks and rest. Complete the movement as a lying down exercise.

Are you ready to make it harder? Please don't try to make it harder. CARs are a feel-good movement designed to keep your joints mobile. We don't want to force them to work harder, just better!

Seated Clock Toe Taps

Clock toe taps as a seated exercise focus on hip mobility, as you straighten and bend your leg, rotating it in the hip socket.

To start: Sit on the edge of a sturdy chair. A dining room chair with no arms is best for optimal movement. Make sure there are no obstacles in a semi-circle in front of you.

Twelve o'clock: Reach your right foot forward with a straight leg and gently tap your big toe at the 12 o'clock position, then return it to the ground beside your left foot.

Moving around the clock: Continue tapping your toe around the imaginary clock, always returning to the center between each "hour" and placing your foot on the ground before continuing to the next "hour."

At the three o'clock position, repeat in the opposite direction, returning to 12 o'clock.

Switch legs: Repeat the toe taps with your left foot, beginning at 12 o'clock and working backward from 11 o'clock down to nine o'clock. Repeat in the opposite direction, returning to 12 o'clock.

Try to do this exercise three times on each side.

Visualize: Imagine that there's a clock face on the floor, and you're standing in the middle of it. The goal is to tap each hour on the clock from 12 o'clock all the way to six o'clock and then repeat the toe taps in the opposite direction back to 12 o'clock.

Do you need to make it easier? If a particular position feels too difficult or uncomfortable, don't reach as far. Instead of tapping the toe on the ground, just lift the leg in that direction and return it to the center, besides your other foot. Start by doing the exercises once on each leg, and gradually work your way up to three repetitions.

Are you ready to make it harder? Repeat this exercise as a standing exercise.

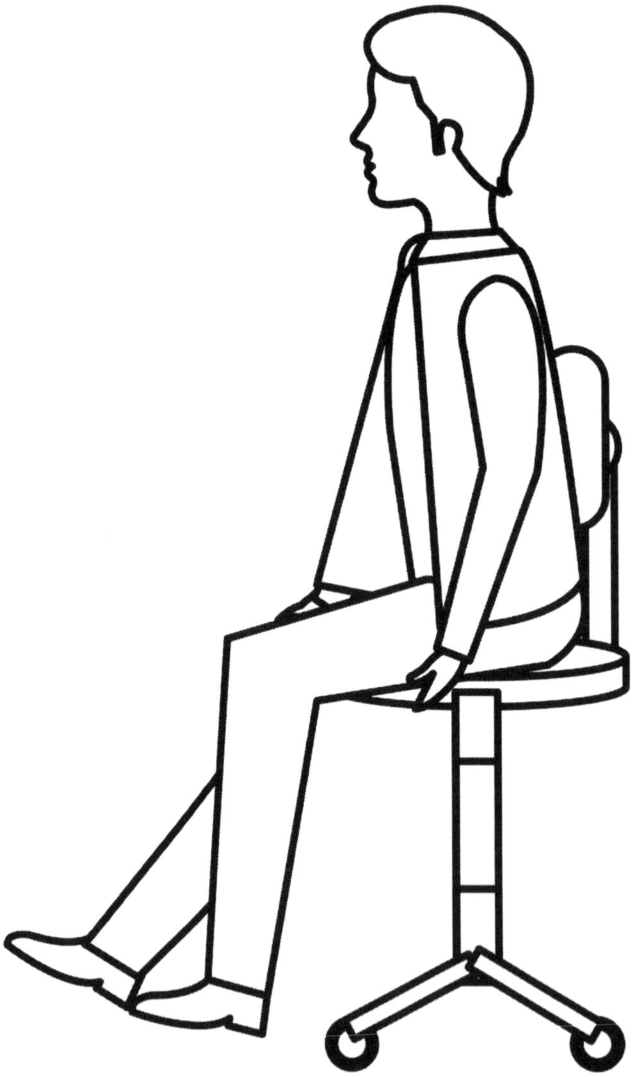

Chapter 7: 4-Week Walking Plan

Walking is one of the most beneficial and simple exercises you can do to stay healthy and fit, so if you've been wondering how to get started or if there's a workout plan that might be appropriate for you, this post is for you. A beginner walking plan and schedule walk through everything from choosing the right shoes to what time of day to walk on what days. If you're looking for a new way to get your daily steps in without having too much trouble with it, keep reading!

Beginner Walking Plan

Walking isn't always an easy activity, especially when it's something new. Like any exercise plan, starting slow will get you to the goal faster.

Here are 6 steps that will help get you started on your walking routine:

1. Decide which type of walking program to follow based on time and speed

If you're looking for a schedule, choose a beginner walking plan. This way, you'll have a set path to follow.

2. Buy the right shoes for your walking workout

Shoes that are comfortable and supportive are necessary to avoid injury when walking for exercise or just when walking around in general. Look into walking shoes when buying new shoes to use during your next walk.

3. Fit your workout into your schedule

Make a habit of walking and make it a regular piece of your daily routine. For example, walk on the way to work or school and on days you don't feel like going to the gym.

4. Decide if you want to walk indoors or outdoors

When it comes to the weather, this is up to you. It's completely fine if you want to walk inside for most of the year and then move outdoors when spring and summer come around. Or, if you want to do the opposite, that's acceptable too!

5. Take a good look at your planner and decide on the days and times you'll walk

Like any exercise routine, consistency is important. Make sure you work out at least 3 to 5 days a week for 30 minutes or more. You can always add more time if it's not hard for you to fit in your workout every day.

6. Monitor your progress

If you want to know if your program is working, try measuring your progress with a pedometer. This will help you see how many steps you're taking each day and let you know if this plan is doing the trick for you!

4-Week Walking Plan

It's a good idea to gradually build up to a longer walking plan, especially if you're a beginner. By doing this slowly, you'll be able to avoid injuries and get the most out of your workout. If you want to start with this beginner walking plan, here are the details:

Week 1

15 minutes of walking 3 times per day until it gets easy.

Week 2

30-minute walks 4 times per day until it gets easy

Week 3

40-minute walks 5 times per day, increasing distance by 10 steps each walk

Week 4

45-minute walks 6 times per day until it becomes easy again!

These are just examples of how to build up an exercise program over time.

Note: You don't need to increase the time every week only progress when it gets easy. Don't push yourself too hard - if you're struggling, take it slow! Every week I like to walk for 30 minutes or more 3–4 times a week for my 30–60 minutes of daily exercise. Don't be afraid to ask friends, coworkers, or anyone that will listen if they'd like to join your morning walks.

How Fast Should You Walk?

So, how fast should you walk?

For beginners, it is recommended to start out with a steady pace that you can hold for 30 minutes or more. This may be a little slow for some people, but it will be beneficial in the long run. Once you get accustomed to this level of intensity and the benefits of it (such as health and fitness) increase faster than your pace, then it is safe to push yourself to walk faster if you would like. Even though the intensity will increase, at first, I recommend you keep your pace at about 75% of max heart rate. Once you're comfortable with this type of training (and see how much progress you're making), then increase the speed that is about 10% each week. At this point, if you'd like to walk faster, it is safe to do.

Gauge your progress!!! If you are not progressing at the pace you are comfortable with, take it slow! Slow down or stop. You can't go back now. There are countless books out there that cover the specifics of every stride pattern/type you will use in your training, which is worth investing in if you're serious about becoming fit and healthy. As with any type of fitness training, it's important to be consistent and build up your resistance level gradually.

Conclusion

There are many women over 60 who exercise for increased strength and fitness, but there is often little guidance on what to do. Strength training should be tailored to the needs of the individual. A woman's physiology can change with age, so it is advisable for women over 60 to take a few things into consideration to ensure safety while exercising. Intensity must not exceed 70% of 1-RM or 8–12 reps; frequency should not exceed 2x/wks.; training sessions should be limited in duration (30 minutes is preferred); and exercises must emphasize big movements rather than stabilizing muscles. Trainers must monitor individuals closely as their perceived exertion will likely decrease over time. If you follow the guidelines of this book, you will be able to exercise safely and effectively for many years.

As you start to age, it is important that you prevent falls by making regular physical activity a part of your daily routine. This will help improve balance and stability so you can stay active for as long as possible.

Staying physically active will not only boost your health but will also improve your overall quality of life as well as boost your mood and energy levels. Take the time to figure out how you can include a balance of moderate aerobic

exercise and strength training each week.

Fortunately, strong is the new sexy! Diverse exercise programs that target all muscle groups can improve strength in older adults just as effectively as regular strength training alone. The problem is that many older adults are unsure of how to incorporate strength training into their workouts due to a lack of knowledge about proper form and technique for this type of exercise. If you are an older adult, it's important that you know how to use proper form so that you don't put your body at risk for injury.

As an older adult, it is common to experience muscle loss and decreased strength due to the amount of activity you participate in. However, strength training exercises can help combat this issue by increasing lean muscle mass. This will help improve balance and stability while also preventing falls.

The goal of most workouts is to increase your heart rate through aerobic exercise for 30 minutes at least five days per week. It is recommended that if you are interested in incorporating strength training into your regimen that you do so after your aerobic workout is complete or on the same day as your cardio session.

Strength training and focus on specific muscle groups can help you improve your overall strength and overall fitness. If you are an older adult, especially if you have osteoporosis, it is important that you incorporate strength training exercises into your routine so that you can prevent falls and increase overall functionality. Strength training by itself is not enough to prevent falls; it is important that they are paired with aerobic exercise for 30 minutes at least five days per week.

While strength training exercises are an important addition to your workout regimen, it is crucial that you pair them with aerobic exercise for 30 minutes at least five days per week. Strength training by itself is simply not enough to prevent falls.

Balance and stability are important factors in preventing falls and thus slowing down the aging process. Strength training exercises can help increase both of these factors, which will help you to prevent falls and remain independent as long as possible.

Strength training exercises will also boost your metabolism and increase lean muscle mass; this can help improve bone density and strength, which is important later in life to prevent osteoporosis.

Strength training exercises aren't just for younger people; they can be effective in improving strength, balance, and stability in older adults who want to remain active into their later years.

As we end this book, here are some guidelines you should remember to stay fit and strong as you begin to feel the aging process:

1. Strength Training

Strength training is essential for most women over 40. If you have no strength training experience, I suggest doing three to four exercises for your hamstrings, quadriceps, lower back and chest twice a week. An exercise program should include 6–12 exercises per muscle group twice a week.

2. Conditioning

Conditioning workouts are more intense than strength workouts and are designed to challenge the system in each workout. You should do conditioning workouts 2-5 times per week for 30–45 minutes per session.

3. Flexibility

The stretching program should be done 4–5 times per week, at least 30 minutes per session. You can also do this type of workout in lieu of a conditioning workout 2–3 times per week for 30 minutes or more.

You may find that you need to work out during the day to keep the workouts fresh and do not have time for a full-time schedule. If you do, remember to make your sessions no more than 45 minutes in duration. The key is to exercise regularly and regularly spaced throughout the week without neglecting any one area for longer periods between workouts.

4. A diet that includes plenty of fresh fruits and vegetables, whole grains, lean proteins, and water throughout the day can help you stay fit as you age.

To keep the body healthy and knowing you're doing the best you can for your physical well-being is always a positive attitude.

I've made it my mission in life to better women's lives through strength training, which is what this book is all about.

5. Exercise Is an Investment in Your Future

Exercise, even when times are tough, helps you cope with life's hard times. If you are unable to exercise because of illness or injury, find a way to do so. You will feel better. You will be happier.

6. Keep in Mind That the Only Goal Is FITNESS

This is an exercise book aimed at older women and for anyone who wants to look and feel better through strength training. No one should have to wait until they are over 60 or 70 years old to feel that they are still in shape or to look fit, regardless of their age.

I hope that this book has given you plenty of ideas and inspiration, such as what to do after your strength training workout and how to start exercising for the very first time.

I hope you've enjoyed this book and will be able to incorporate these techniques into your lifestyle. The path to optimal health and fitness is fun and easy when you know what exercises to do and how, but it can also be challenging if you don't know what exercises not to do.

Thank you for this wonderful opportunity and for purchasing this book. I hope you discover the joys of strength training and look forward to more information and advice in the future.

Printed in Great Britain
by Amazon

70367018R00070